The Building of

"Courage"

ISBN-10: 0615400027   ISBN-13: 978-0-615-40002-0

The Building of

"*Courage*"

A sculpture standing in tribute to those
who have, who are, and who will battle Cancer

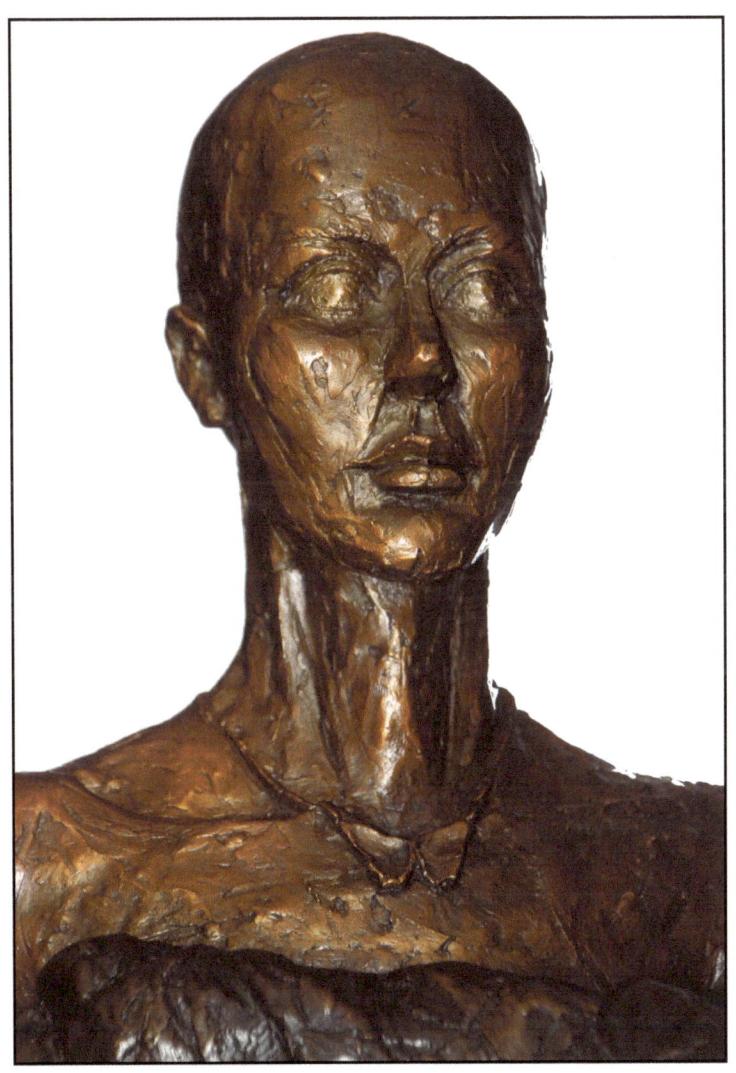

By Artist Michael L. Tieman

Published by

Michael Tieman Publishing

PO Box 1326,

Cannon Beach, OR

97110, USA

www.courageforcancer.net

E-mail: mt@courageforcancer.net

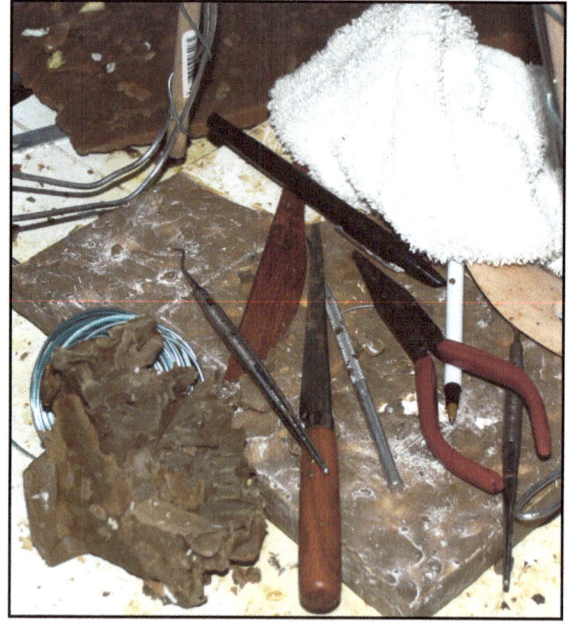

Printed in U.S.A.

First Printing April 2009

Dedicated to the women in my family

who have battled breast cancer;

my mother-in-law Janet Ormandy Marshall (Muzzy),

my aunt Pat Wetzel,

my sister Beverly Starr,

and my younger sister

Connie Sue Drotos,

who after a courageous six year battle

with breast cancer,

died on July 29, 2008.

Always a positive attitude and a smile

Muzzy and Connie were an inspiration

to those battling breast Cancer,

and they will be sorely missed.

The Dream . . .

"In July of 2008, after a courageous six year battle with breast cancer, my younger sister died, one week shy of her 50th birthday and the day before her 25th wedding anniversary," says Tieman. "Since then I have had the same re-occurring dream. I am on a scaffold built around a piece of white marble 15' tall, and I am carving a figure titled 'Courage' – she has a bald head wrapped in cloth, piercing eyes, a firm jaw, taunt body and feet apart yet firmly planted. The people battling cancer have an inner strength and courage as they not only face an uncertain future, but they also have to take their treatments knowing it will make them feel worse. Yet, week after week they look forward to this pain in hopes it will eventually be gone. There is a look of courage in their eyes I cannot describe with words, it's not entirely defiant (Cancer will not win), but actually shows a grace with a quiet determination. That is the courage I need to capture.

In the dream I can only sense the figure; all I can really see is the head. I am carving with a chisel and hammer, no power tools. I can see my scarred swollen hands and feel the pain in them as I continuously strike the chisel. Yet, there are many unanswered questions; why is the stone exactly 15' tall, why can't I see the entire figure? I am carving the stone by looking at a maquette of the piece, but how do I know it is exactly 36" tall since I can only see the head?

I have begun the 36" tall maquette, born from wire and pipe and clay. Starting with the bald head, piercing eyes and a heart in the courageous chest, and yet I know the face is not that of my sister. And someday I hope I will get a commission to begin the final piece, carved out of a 15' block of pure white marble, 'Courage', standing in tribute to those who have, who are, and who will battle Cancer."

The Promise ...

"People who saw me building the clay sculpture 'Courage', November 8th and 9th during my demo at the 2008 Stormy Weather Arts Festival at Haystack Gallery in Cannon Beach, Oregon expressed a need for the piece to be seen and touched ... now. So I am casting 'Courage' in a limited edition bronze in three sizes, 9 foot high heroic size, 36" high and 18" high maquettes. With up to half of the sale price being donated directly to a local hospital or Cancer center's Cancer Support Services. These support services offer daily comfort and support to patients battling Cancer. This book The Building of 'Courage' which originally was to be made to accompany each sculpture will now also be published in a larger quantity for people who want the book so they can be connected to 'Courage'.

'Courage' has found her destiny, and this is the story of the journey she has taken for all of us."

July 29, 2008

Grabbing the first flight out of Portland, Oregon this morning, I arrive at the Chicago airport around noon. I am on my way to be at the bedside of my younger sister, Connie Sue, who is in a hospital in Akron Ohio, dying of Cancer. While running to my next plane connection to Cleveland, I turn on my cell phone and it chimes with a voice message to be picked up. Dreading the message, I see it is from my sister, Beverly, who is already at the hospital along with Connie's husband John, and our dad. I stop at the nearest empty gate waiting area and sit down to hear the message, knowing in my heart that I did not make it in time to be with Connie one last time, that she is already gone.

August 5

Nancy, my wife of 36 years and I came back home from Connie's funeral in Akron on Sunday the 3rd. Today would have been Connie's 50th birthday. She died, one day before John and her 25th wedding anniversary, and a week before this her 50th birthday. This is a sad, lonely day for the family, especially for John.

August 6

I had the strangest dream last night. This is what I hauntingly remember…

I am on a scaffold built around a piece of white marble 15' tall, and I am carving a figure titled "Courage" – she has a bald head wrapped in cloth, piercing eyes, a firm jaw, taunt body and feet apart yet firmly planted. I can only sense the figure; all I can really see is the head.

August 14

Every night since the 5th I have had the beginning of the same dream. Some nights like last night more has been revealed to me.

In the dream I can only sense the figure; all I can really see is the head. I am

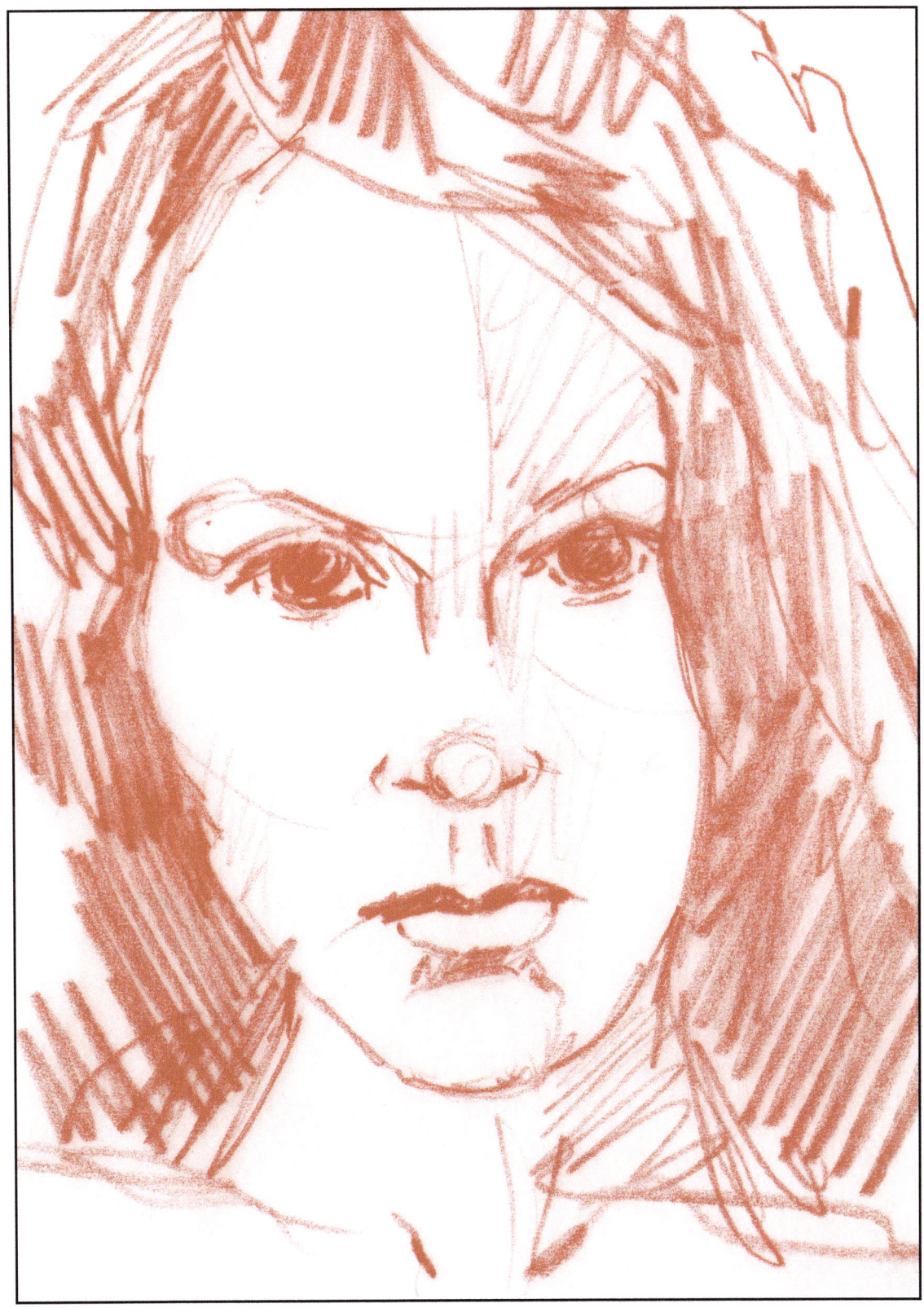

carving with a chisel and hammer, no power tools. I can see my scarred swollen hands and feel the pain in them as I continuously strike the chisel.

What does this all mean? Is this dream from deep inside of me, or coming from Connie? Something she left unfinished, or a task she has left for me? There are many unanswered questions; why is the stone exactly 15' tall, why can't I see the entire figure, I am carving the stone by looking at a maquette of the piece, but how do I know it is exactly 36" tall since I can only see the head?

August 15

Still haunted nightly by the dream, I have tried to sketch out the head and face, but to no avail. Nothing I draw is right. The power of the vision eludes me. Yet I continue to draw hoping to find it. Every piece I have ever worked on, paintings or sculptures all have started as an idea in my head that I have developed on paper by drawing it out. But this piece I can't seem to draw and I have never had a piece continually invade my dreams.

August 16

Again with the dream. I have seen it enough now to be able to piece together in my mind the look.

People battling Cancer have an inner strength and courage as they not only face an uncertain future, but also have to take their treatments knowing it will make them feel worse, yet week after week they look forward to this pain in hopes it will eventually be gone. There is a look of courage in their eyes I cannot describe with words, it's not entirely defiant (Cancer will not win), but actually shows a grace and a quiet determination. That is the courage I need to capture.

Sept 23

After more than a month having this same dream, I decided to tell Nancy tonight, being a therapist it's difficult to say what she thinks, maybe I am crazy. She went to bed before me and came running out of the bedroom in her bed shirt. "This is how I see her standing", she said, and stood straight up, head held high, chest out, feet apart and arms swung back with clenched fists. "Here and

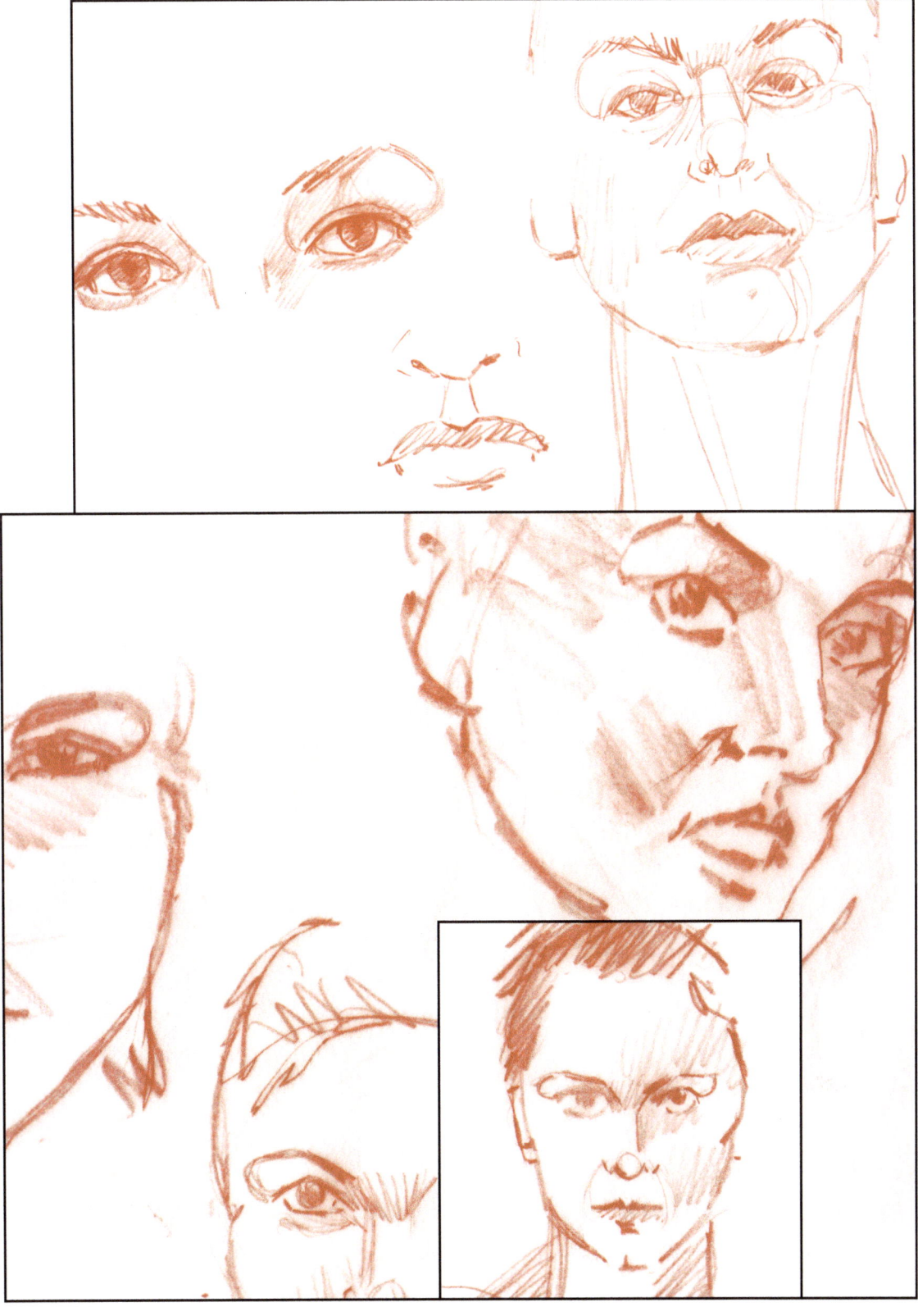

no further, the line in the sand." For the first time I can see the figure developing. My soul mate and partner has started the process as she sees "Courage". This dream of mine is beginning to take shape, beginning to get a life of her own, beginning to affect the thoughts of others. Is this what "Courage" is meant to do? Is she to become her own self outside of my vision?

Sept 25

Still the dream every night, I can delay no longer. I need a restful night's sleep. Today I have begun "Courage". I went to the local hardware store and bought the pipe, wire, and wood to start the armature. 1" galvanized pipe with elbow and "t" joints, ¼" dowels for support and a white board to become the base. I spent the afternoon cutting and building the wood base, connecting the pipe and wrapping the 14' of 9 gauge wire to form the inside armature support. Formed the wire head and hip cages and added the dowels to the wire for additional support to hold the weight of the clay. She takes life, held together with wire and wood and metal pipe. My vision is taking form.

Sept 26

I have started to shape the head and face, but my first act is to place a heart in the chest of "Courage". This is something I have done since my very first sculpture back in 2003. I read an article about a woman sculptor who always started this way, placing a heart shape in the chest of each of her sculptures. She said it brought the piece to life; it gave the sculpture not only a heart, but a soul as well. So I use it as well, and it has worked.

Sept 27

I begin the head and face in the classic style and proportions. The head is 1/8th the height of the body to the ankles, and the width of the head from center of the nose to outer edge at the eyes is 1/3 the head height. The head is divided in thirds again from the top of the head to the bottom of forehead, from there to the bottom of nose and from there to the bottom of chin. The eyes divide the head in half from top to bottom. The width of the nose is equal to the width of the eye, and the eyes are one eye apart. Width of lips is from the center of one eye to the center of

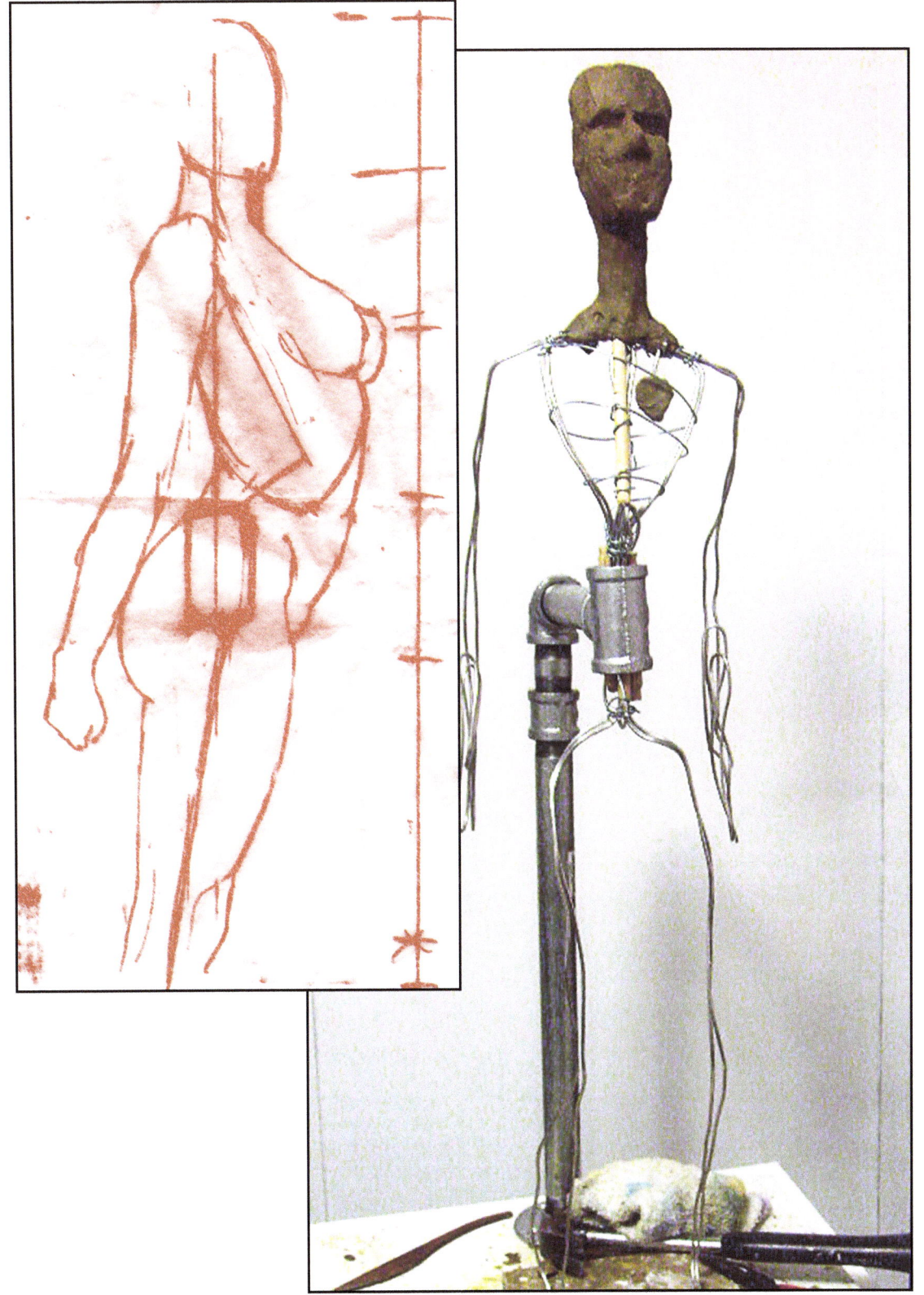

the other, and the bottom of the lips divide the lower face from bottom of nose to chin in half. The width of a lady's neck and the length from chin to sternum is ½ head. All very math oriented, and I use these measurements only as a reference to begin building. Then I build and sculpt from there.

Oct 3

Each night I have worked on the face, and the eyes, thinking I have it right. And the next night I redo them. The face is one of my "ladies". Strong chiseled jaw, and high cheekbones, but it's the eyes. I have never added the eyes to my sculptures because I want the entire piece to be seen as the expression of the movement. But now it is more than the movement and body, it is in the eyes I have to succeed.

Oct 5

Today I started a news release to announce my new sculpture, "Courage". I have written and re-written it about a dozen times. The message needs to be there clearly communicated without being sappy. I have also decided to take Patty (co-owner of Haystack Gallery), up on her offer to be a part of the Cannon Beach Stormy Weather Arts Festival by working on "Courage" in Haystack Gallery in Cannon Beach on Sunday, Nov. 9.

Oct 6

There has been a discussion between my oldest daughter, Heather, and Nancy about whether "Courage" should have breasts. My sculptures, with women, are all well endowed, and Heather objects strongly to having breasts on "Courage". So many women who have battled breast cancer have had mastectomies, losing one or both breasts. I must confess, I did not even think about it. It does make sense, but what about those women who have had reconstructive surgery? Or none like Connie? How to represent all?

The more I ponder, the more obvious it becomes. Instead of having both arms at the side and slightly behind in a stance of defiance, I will move one arm forward and cover her breasts. But, the arm doesn't cover enough. By adding a cloth

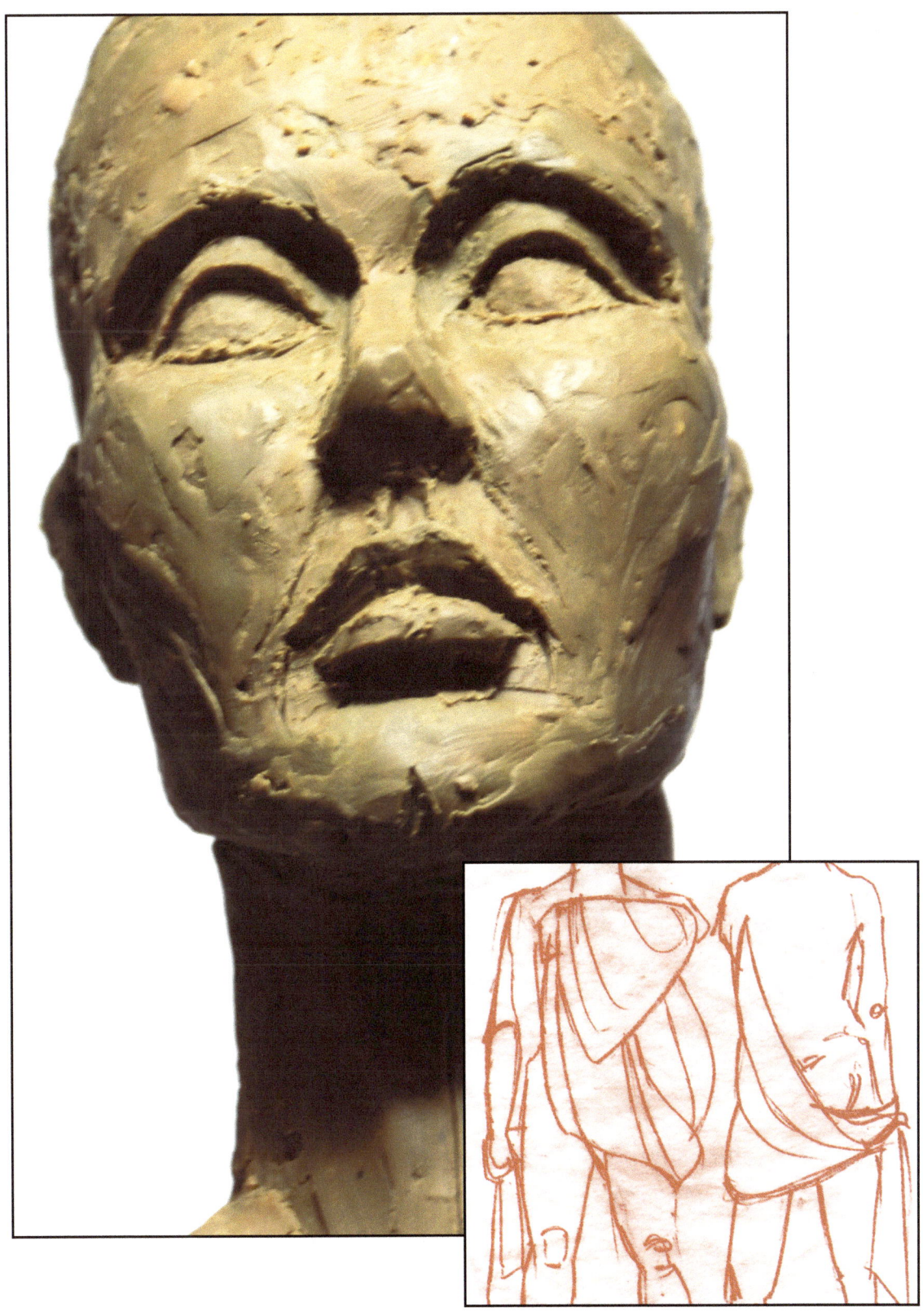

that covers the chest and folds over the arm, you can't tell if she has breasts or not.

Interesting this move causes "Courage" to look as though she is holding up the cloth as a shield, covering while also protecting, as though a warrior going into battle. The stance of the body is starting to come together, and a warrior needs a sword to go with the shield. By wrapping the cloth around her back, and holding the cloth bunched and draped in her right hand with some of the cloth falling down, it looks like she is holding a sword.

This is looking very promising. It adds a more defined and focused message. It also allows the cloth to not only symbolize these things, but it also will soften the severity of the figure. Additionally it allows a device for movement of the form and helps move your eyes around the figure. From the mouths of kids comes simple understanding.

Oct 8

I sent a draft of the news release to my sister Beverly to make sure the information was accurate. Her response was unexpected, since I said that the face of "Courage" was not Connie's. And then she sent the email on to her daughter, Amy.

"I think this is beautiful. It's not Connie's face because there are just so many fighters and survivors out here. I understand."

"I think this is one of the most beautiful things I have ever read. I can picture the woman just as you describe her. Thank you for sharing your dream - I will treasure this always.

"Courage" it seems has taken on a life of her own. Another surprise from Beverly. She has decided to leave Richardson, Texas to visit Cannon Beach for the Stormy Weather Arts Festival and see Nancy and me and this sculpture she has heard about. Bev hates flying and in 35 years has never been to the west

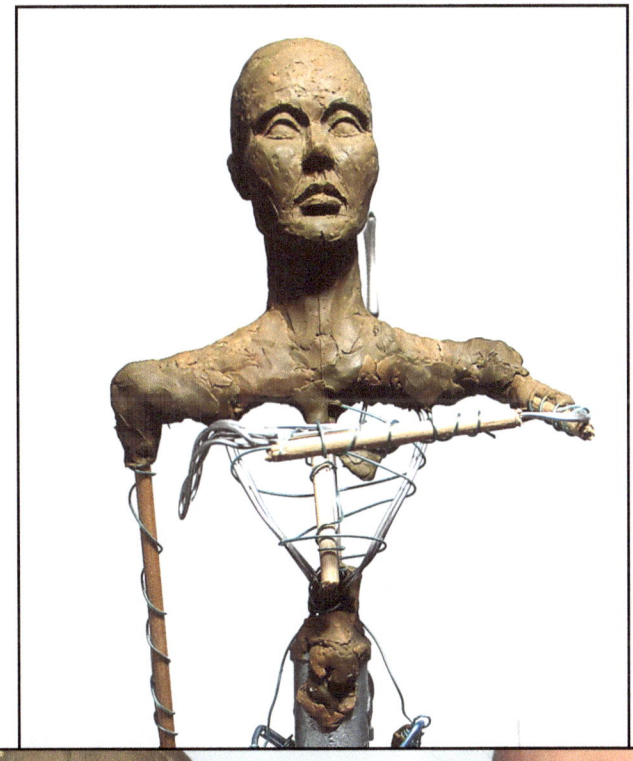

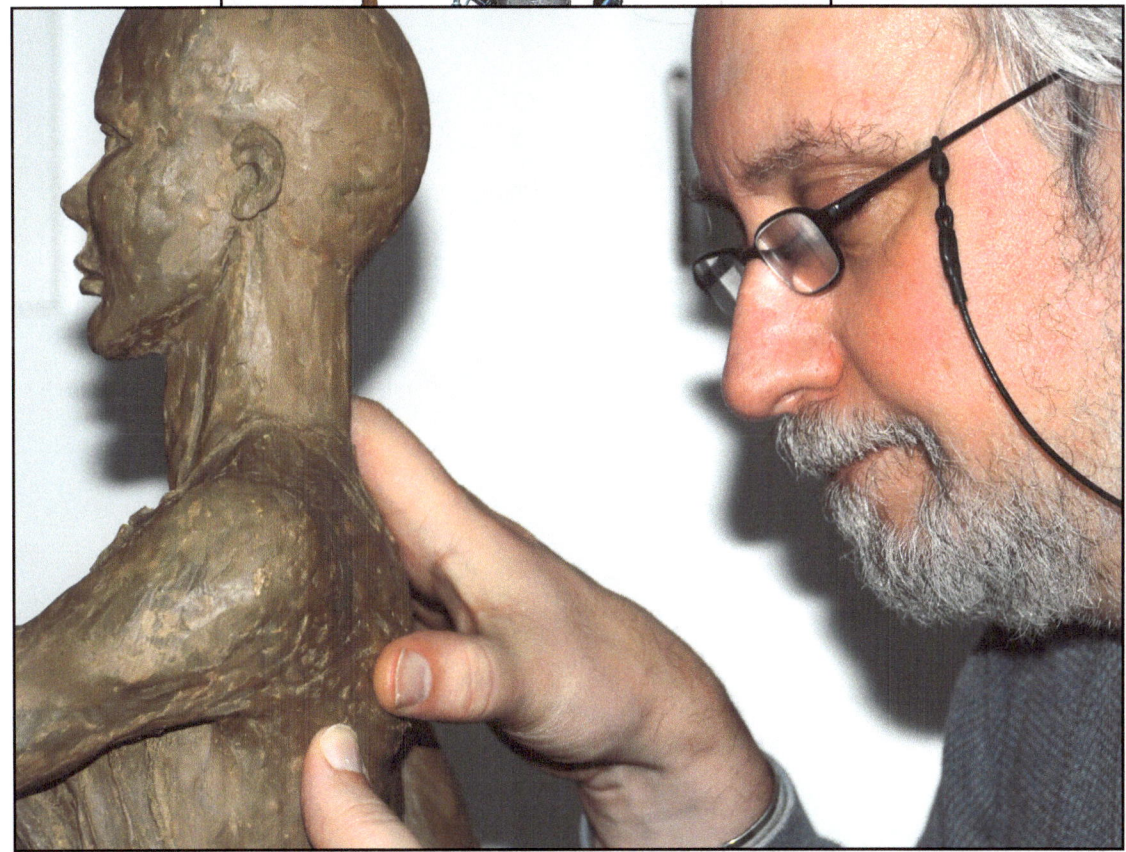

coast to see us. Says she has never seen me work before, nor seen any of my paintings or sculptures in person and this seems the perfect time to do so. I think she is coming to see if I am as crazy as I sound. It will be great to see her and introduce her to our friends and quaint little town. She will be here over a week, should have some fun.

Oct 9

Now the final test, I am sending out the release to family and friends.

"I'm so sorry to learn about your sister. I knew that she was ill, and I'm sad to know that she lost the battle. Breast cancer has touched so many of my friends and relatives. And what a wonderful tribute you are working on. It will be interesting to watch it unfold and to eventually know why it is 15' high. I have the feeling from your message that this is a "torturing" project in many ways for you … it is going to be a challenging journey. Thank you for taking it for all of those it will honor."

"It is incredibly meaningful work you are doing —plus, your words from the press release are so moving. Perhaps we could include them in the story? There is nothing I could write that would be more powerful."   – Cannon Beach Gazette

A feature story in the local newspaper. It seems "Courage" has become her own woman and is meant to be shared with the world. The 36" clay maquette will be cast in bronze. I don't know how I will find the money, or how many there will be in the limited edition, but she will happen.

Oct 12

Sent the release out to the press, now I wait to see if there is any interest.

Oct 13

Out of the blue I received a phone call today from the Director of Marketing at a local hospital. The Daily Astorian newspaper sent him my news release and he had to call me. The story touched him so much since his mother and father had

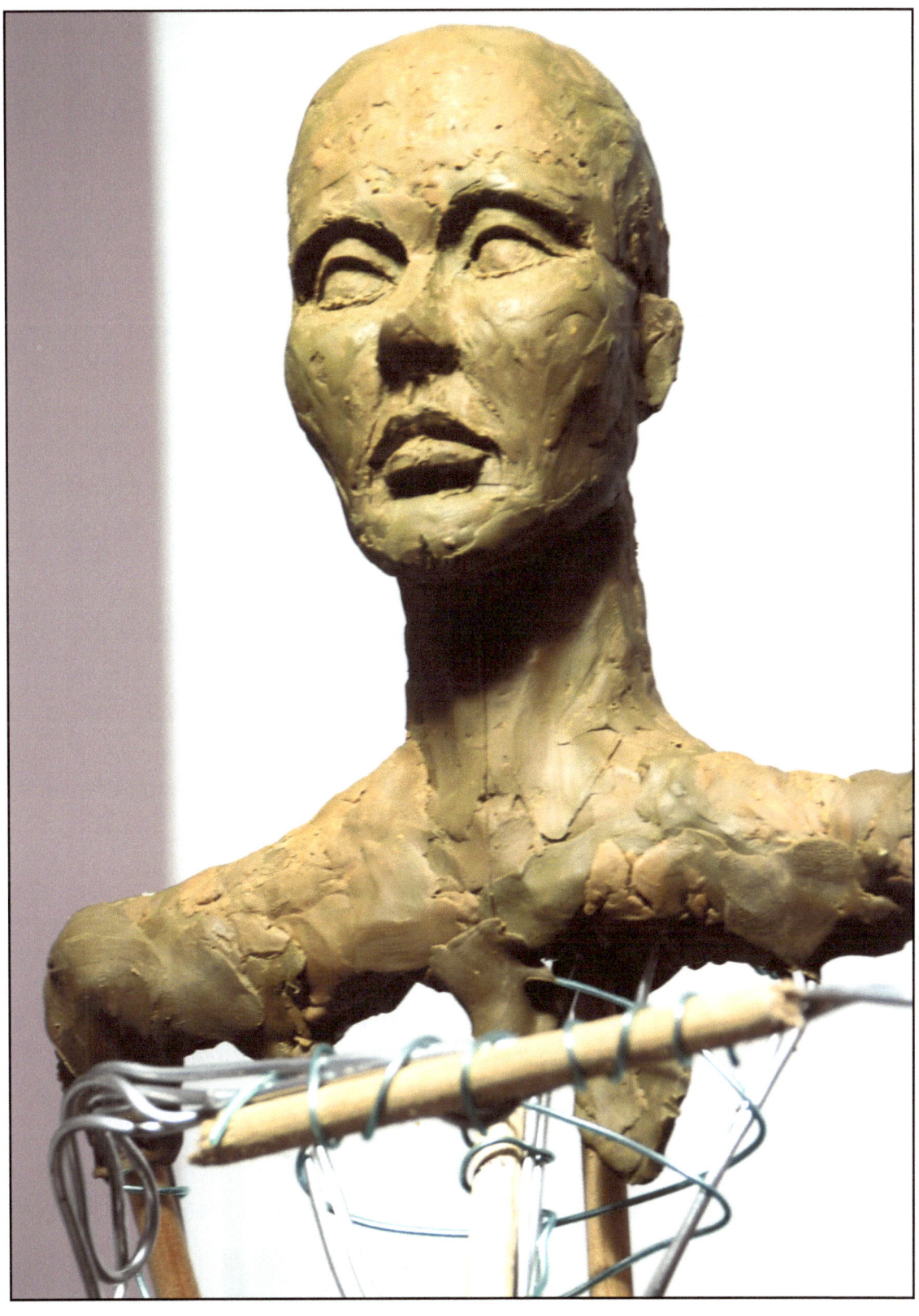

Cancer. The just of it was, what could they do to for me and vice versa? It was a touching conversation and a hard one for me. I am not use to sharing my emotions like this; I am a very private and introverted person.

Oct 14

Called and emailed the Burning Palace foundry in Boring, Oregon to get prices on the 36" and an 18" "Courage". The ones I sell direct I can give half to charity. If it is sold in a gallery, the gallery will only get 25% and the other 25% will go to charity. Now to decide which charity for cancer organization gets the money. I want the money to go directly to the patients to make their treatments a bit better, for chairs, or art, or iPods, or a TV. This is what "Courage" is all about. Not the research or the fundraising for new centers, but to improve the surroundings and amenities on a day to day basis. There has to be a national organization set up to take money for this.

Oct 21

Asked for mold and casting prices on "Courage" earlier in the week and was able to get them today, in time for my meeting with the hospital. I was pleasantly surprised with the prices; I thought they would come in higher. I have worked with the foundry for the last six years, and they understand me and what I want. Now the sculptures become more affordable with the charity still making good money.

Oct 24

I had my first meeting today with the hospital. We discussed the 3' tall piece and how many in the limited edition. I originally thought about 150. Nancy thinks more than a couple of hundred and the marketing director thinks that if it goes national we should be thinking of thousands. Then discussed the smaller, 18" size, same thing with editions, and Steve kept coming back to a large "Courage" in the courtyard the hospital is building. I explained that the 15' marble piece would be very expensive. It would be 45 tons of marble, quarried in Italy at a cost of just the stone to be around $200,000. A commission of this would be at least $1.5 million, with half going to charity. The idea came up to do an edition

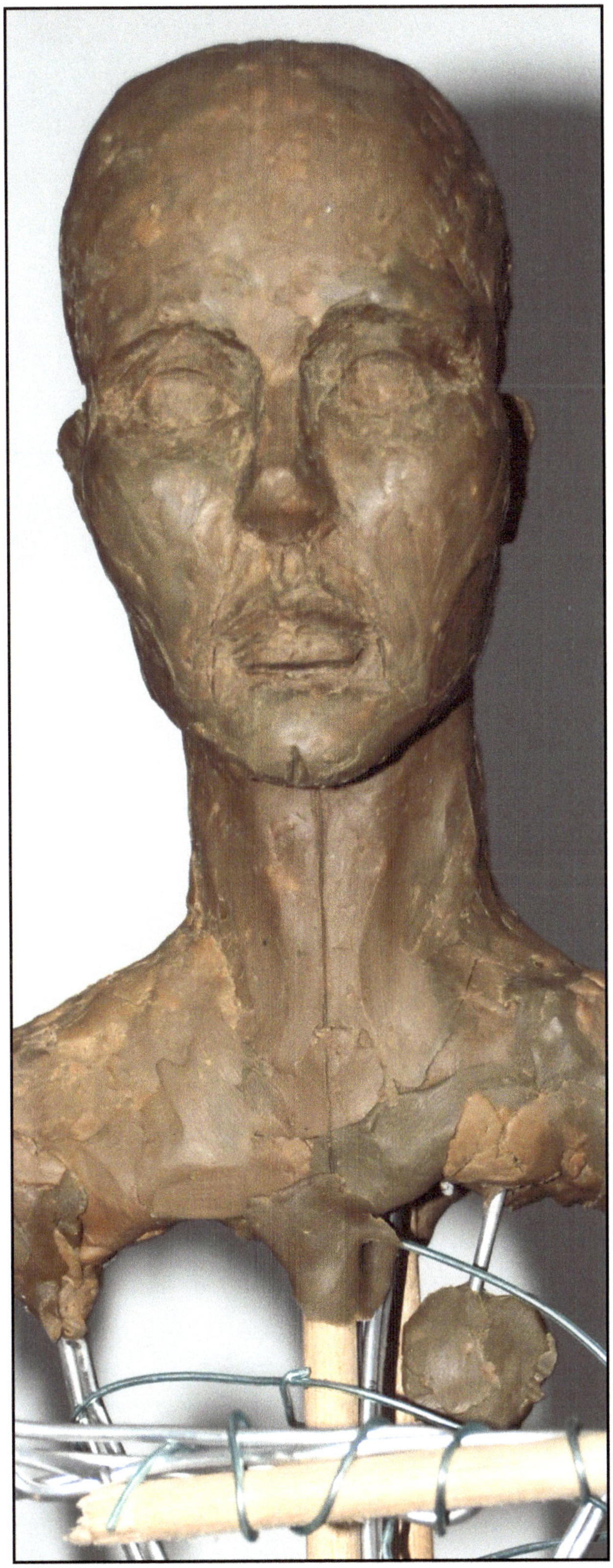

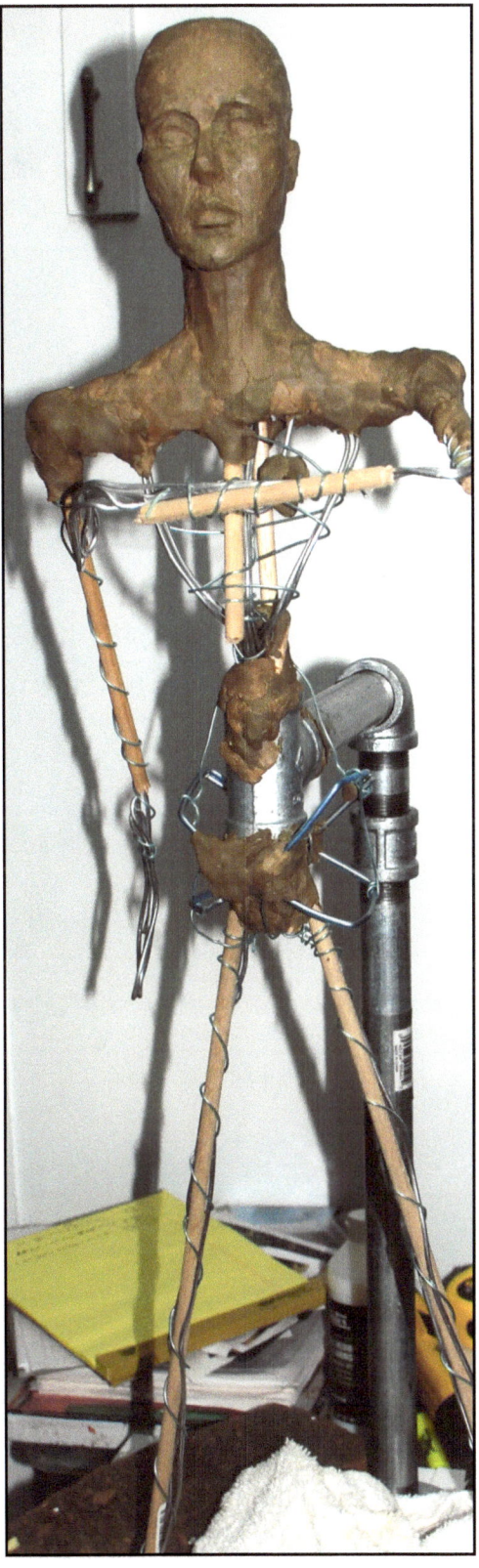

of a heroic size 9' bronze for hospitals and clinics to buy for their facilities. Also discussed the idea I had about doing a book on the entire process of the building of "Courage"; from initial drawings to photos of the piece under construction to the photos of it being completed at the foundry. I thought it would be a nice book that went with the sculpture so the buyers could see how it was made. Steve thought a DVD should also be made, and both sold by themselves. That way those who could not afford the sculpture could be connected to the piece through the book or DVD. Also the butterfly necklace (Connie loved butterflies) and bracelet (that I had made for my family with the inscription Love Never Fails on "Courage" could be sold. There is a fine line between a limited piece of art and over merchandising. I will have to really think this over. But I do realize that all of these items need to be protected by copyright so no one else can produce them.

These ramblings on paper will become the basis for the book ... The Building of "Courage". The time is now for a better digital camera ... maybe a new Nikon.

Oct 30

My new Nikon digital camera came in today. I bought it with some of my inheritance money from my great aunts Maggie & Thelma. I will be using it to document the building of "Courage". Took some shots of the head ... it is good to have a Nikon in my hands again. The quality and feel of the camera and the images live up to what I expect from a Nikon and its controls are similar to my old F4. See the results at right. Large hi-res files (300dpi @ 16"), nice and crisp.

Nov 1

A lady came into the gallery today, drawn in by my sculpture "Spirit of the Sea". She loved the passion, power and grace of the piece. As we talked, I showed her the "Hands of the Artists" collection and she asked what my new piece was. I told her "Courage" and gave her the post card with the story on the back. While she was reading it, tears came to her eyes. After she finished, she came around the counter and hugged me, giving me her condolences and saying she will keep an eye on the progress of the piece via our web site. Then left saying

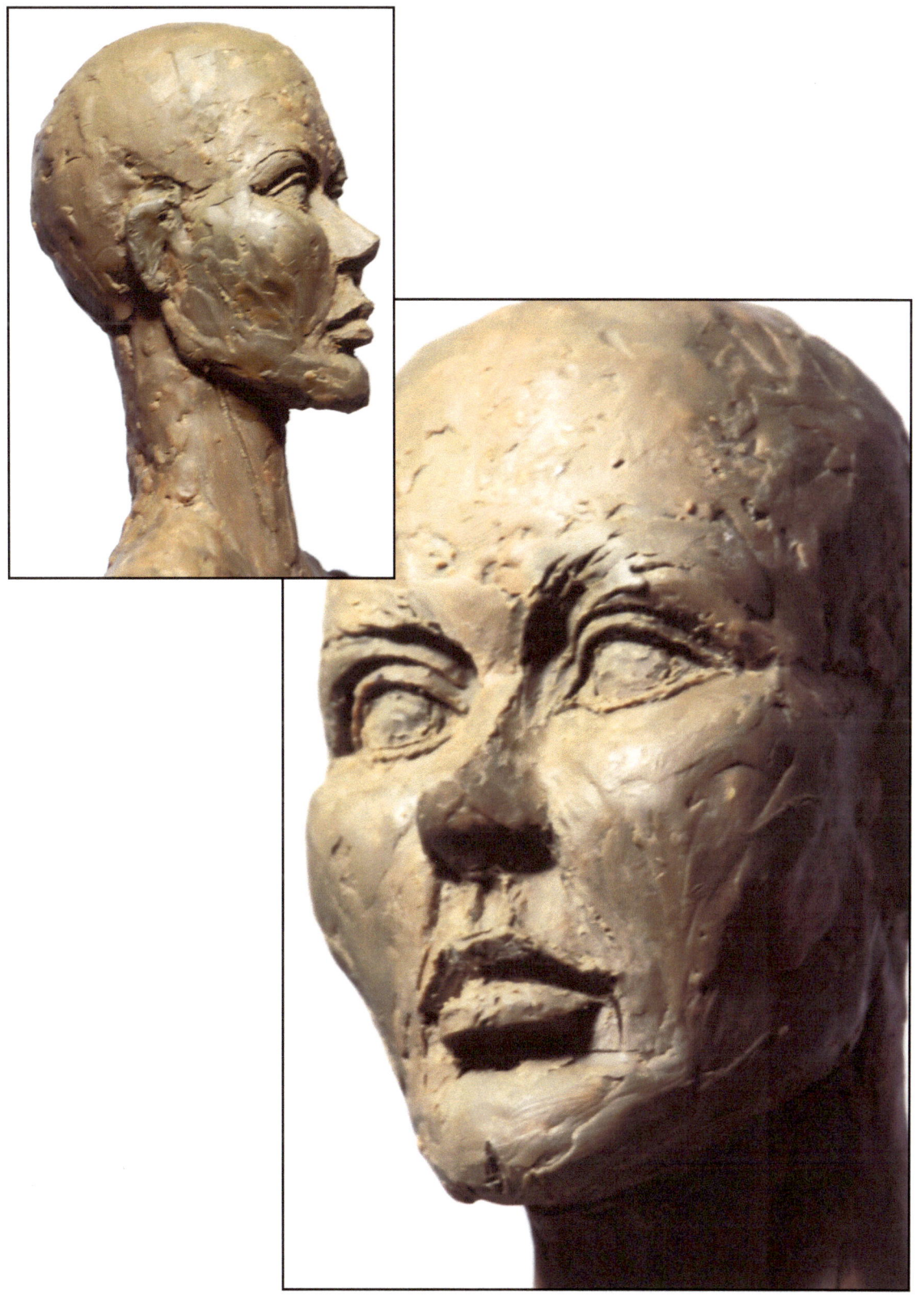

don't be surprised if I see her again soon. I only hope the completed bronze of "Courage" lives up to expectations, and that she is as powerful and emotionally charged as her story.

Nov 3

Tonight I have reworked the eyes yet again, adding more detail in the eyelids and eyebrows and more padding in the eye socket above the eyes. Also added a bit more volume to the cheeks below the cheekbone filled out her face and made it less stark, a bit softer more feminine. She is starting to look more like I think she needs to.

Nov 5

Nancy and I went into Portland tonight to pick up my sister, Beverly who flew in from Dallas to see us, and we spent the night in a hotel in Portland.

Nov. 6

We had dinner with all of our kids and grandkids. Brought Beverly to Cannon Beach, she walked into the house and saw "Courage", but said nothing. Later she said it was too emotional, she couldn't bring herself to speak.

Nov. 7

Spent the day discussing "Courage" with Beverly and showing her my studio, explaining the clay sculpting process and then showing her the stone sculptures I am working on. I spent the rest of the day re-working "Courage", because her head is bald, I need to re-sculpt it so it does not look harsh. Made the back of the head smaller, elongated the jaw, added some fat around the eyes, gave her more eyelids, and added a bit more fat to her cheeks under the cheekbone. I then made her neck a bit thinner and longer, all of this to soften her harshness the bald head made evident. I took "Courage" into Haystack Gallery, getting her ready for her debut this weekend.

Nov. 8

"Courage" was unveiled to the public today. I was supposed to work the gallery,

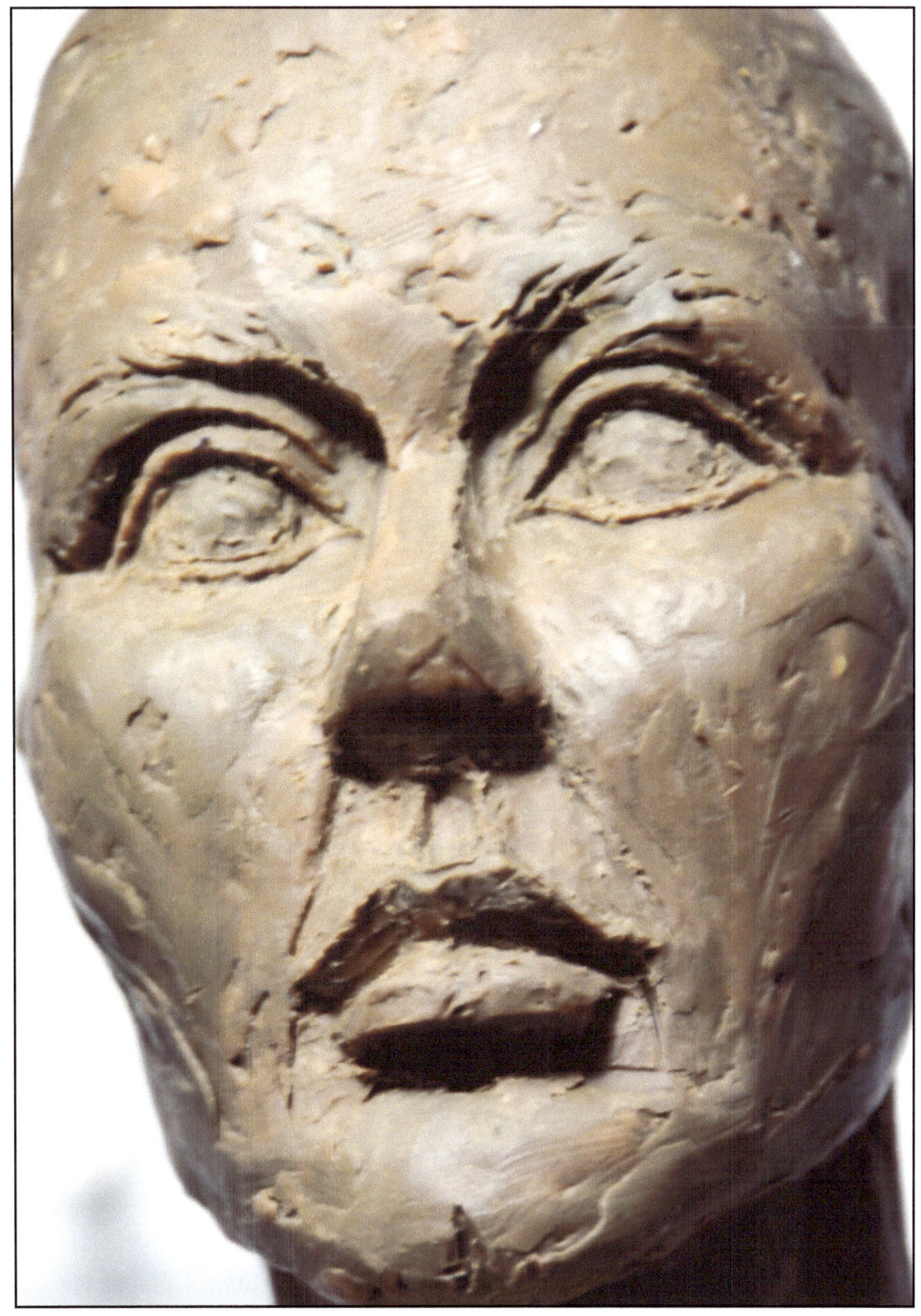

especially since we had a watercolorist doing a demo in the gallery today. We had a gallery full of his groupies, but around it all and after he left, "Courage" was the star attraction, so I spent my time discussing her more than I anticipated. Had a lot of people in who also talked about their experiences, and losses, a multiple Kleenex day. Several other very positive things came out about the piece. The eyes and face are right!!! There were two women in the crowd that came up and shared, one was a breast Cancer survivor of twenty years and her brother recently died of Cancer, and she saw him in the face, and the other woman recently lost her mother to Cancer and she saw her in the face. A connection has been made across gender lines, and both agreed the face/eyes were right. I was talking to a friend and his wife, and tears were coming down his cheeks as we discussed the piece, his wife is a recent breast Cancer survivor. It was still very emotional for him, but the strength he saw in "Courage" was not as the warrior, but that she had the eyes and presence of command, not just the warrior, but the Commander in the battle. He then brought up the fact that the warrior stance is feet apart and firmly planted, but on the balls of their feet and the knees slightly bent. That way they can stand solid and unwavering for a long time. "Courage" has transcended to a higher place and purpose, she is definitely no longer mine, but she is for all.

Nov. 9

Today I was suppose to work on "Courage" in the gallery, a sculpture demo, but it turned into a lot more. I was "holding court", as people were standing, sitting on the floor in front of me, and seated on the stairs completely covering them. And it seemed each of the three groups came in and left to make room for the next. Nothing was scheduled, but it was like clockwork. I explained the dream and the building of the sculpture from the beginning armature through to the piece as it was and then into the foundry part. To re-enforce yesterdays, comments, a lady said she saw "everyone" in the face, and another man spoke of the warrior stance again and how you can stand forever like that. It seems the making the book available to all is a great idea. "Courage" is a piece that seems to help the healing of those who have gone through or are going through Cancer treatments and those left watching their friends and loved ones. Our youngest daughter,

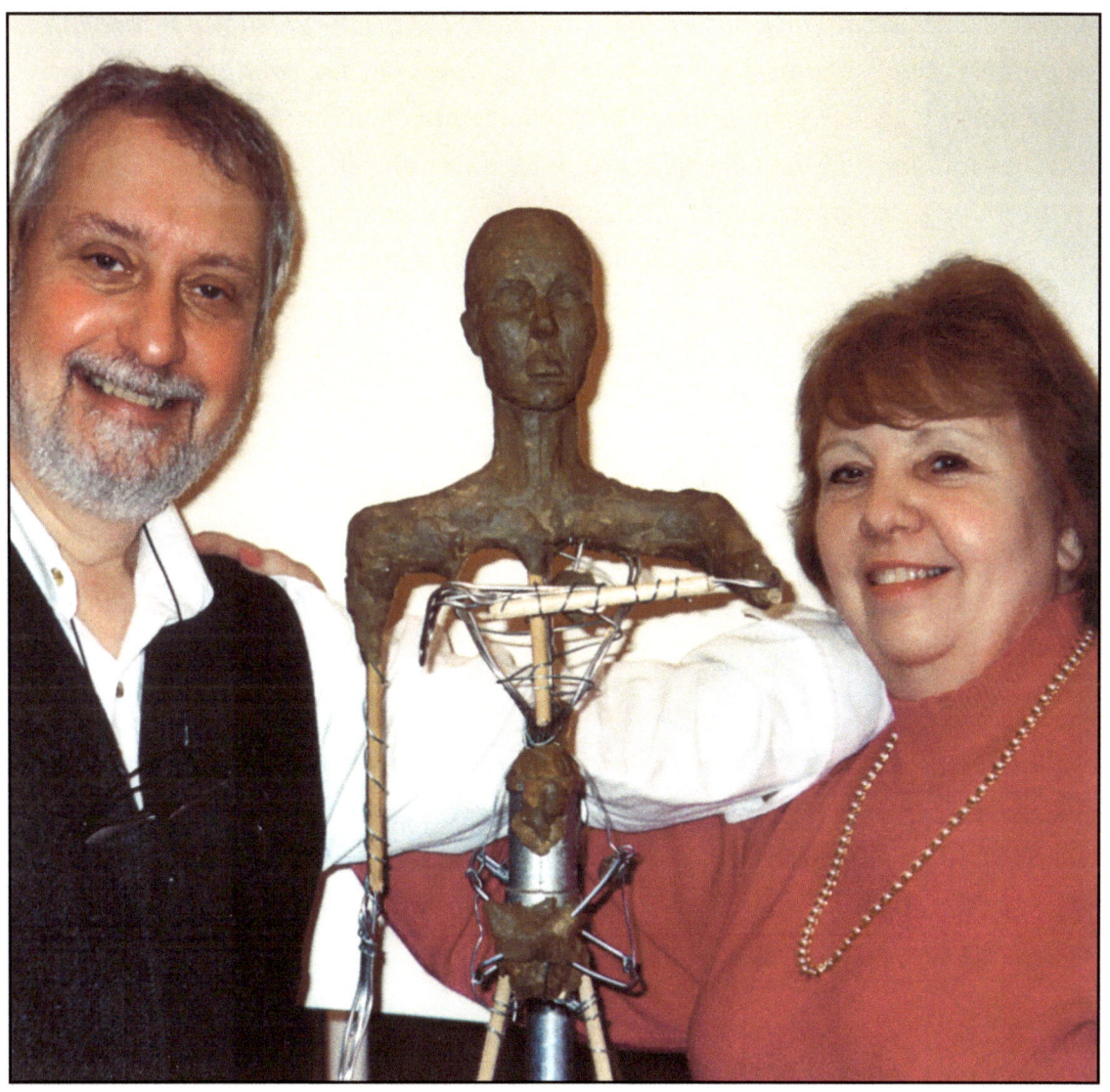

Katie came over from Portland and brought her kids, so they could be here for the show, and at the end of the night she asked a very profound question from one so young, "You as the artist are not in control anymore with what "Courage" will look like. Are you OK with that?" After a moment I explained I was never in charge, the dream or whoever made me start the piece guided my hands in the beginning, and now others are guiding them, I am just the conduit. Unlike my other work, I was never in control, and yes, I am OK with that on this piece. I was and still am surprised by the reaction of others and the power that "Courage" seems to have. It has brought out the softer more emotional side of me which also surprised me. But Nancy says she never doubted what would happen and is surprised I opened myself to all of this. Thus the power of art as a healer…

Steve, a friend of mine since the old days when I was in advertising, came to the show with his fiancé, and we discussed the marketing side of this and should I set up a foundation or non profit or not for profit to make sure the money trail is handled correctly? It is important that "Courage" is not taken advantage of by others. She and the people she touches have to be protected. Her image cannot get tarnished, and the monies raised have to go where they are needed.

Nov. 14

Today I took my sister Beverly to the airport in Portland to go back home to Dallas. While she was here, I sprayed expandable foam on "Courage". This is done to add volume to the piece without the weight of clay. Tomorrow night I will start carving and roughing up the foam in order to begin layering the clay over it. She looks like she has on bib overalls.

Nov. 15

Started to add the oil based clay to the foam structure today, this is my least favorite part as it doesn't take talent, just time and patience. I think the figure is fairly well set now, just small changes to the stance as she develops.

Nov 20 - 21

I finally completed the covering of the foam with clay; "Courage" will now start to take her final shape. This part is where my years of anatomy lessons and

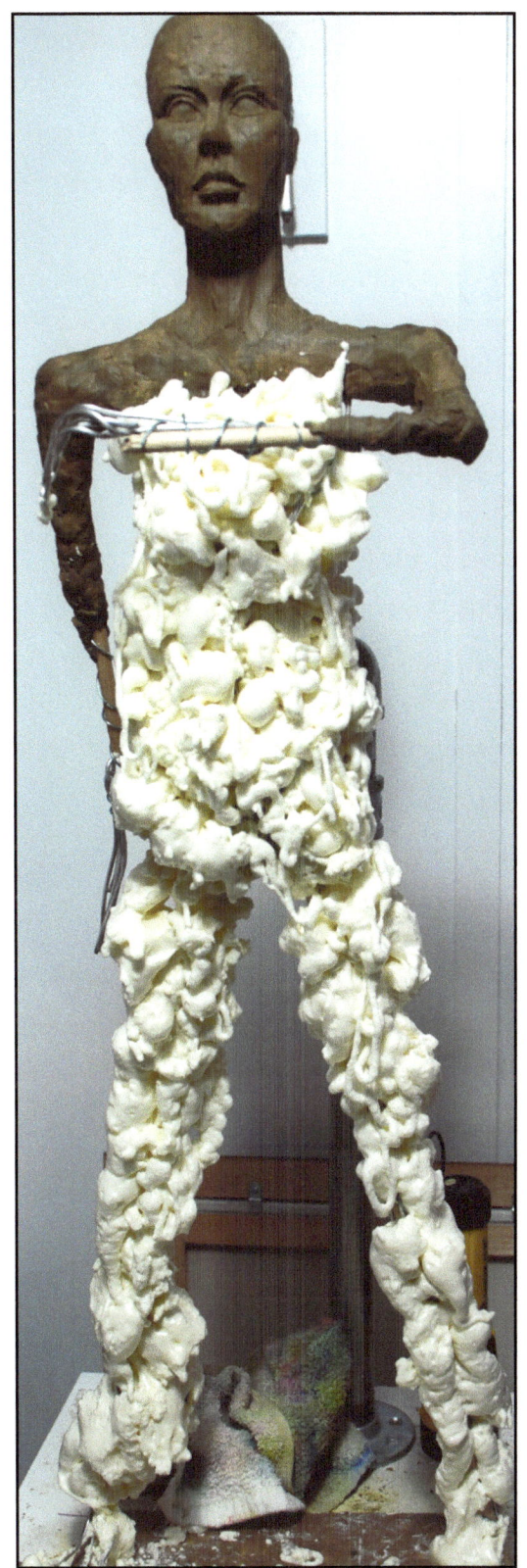
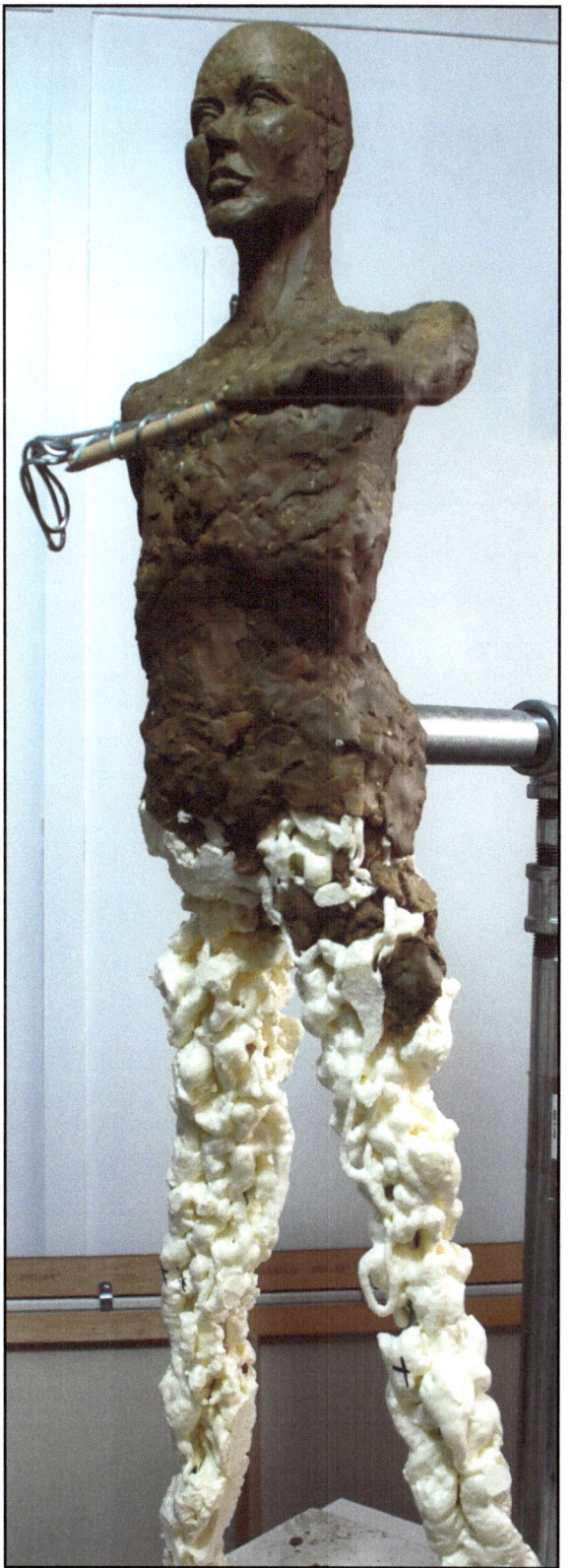

drawing of the figure pay off. I start by putting markers on the clay that show the depth of the clay build-up. Just like CSI, when they reconstruct what the face will look like from just the skull, I start by drawing the main skeletal forms in the clay. Using calipers and a knife, I measure the first large form, the rib cage, using the head as the base measure. The size of all parts of the body is based on the head. I have always made the body Michelangelo's classic eight heads high; this adds more to the length of the legs, making the figure look more elegant and less squatty. Some artists use 7½ heads to 9 heads so there really isn't a standard. By using the eight heads, the main body markers are easy to determine without a lot of math. Taking the head height measurement, and working down the body, the sternum begins ½ head down from the chin, the nipples are one head down from the chin, the belly button another head below the nipples, the crouch a head from the belly button, the knee is two heads from the crouch and the ankles are two heads from the knees. On the female, the waist is about 1 head wide, the hips at the widest point are two heads, and the shoulders are 1½ heads wide to the outside edges, on a male these last two measurements are reversed.

I begin with the construction of the rib cage, the side at its longest is 1½ heads, sternum length is ⅓ head, and the rib cage at its widest (at ribs 7 & 8) is 1½ heads. I measure and draw the rib cage shape on the front, back and both sides with the knife point.

Next I move to the next large form and bone, the hips. Hip bone starts ½ head from the base of the rib cage, and is the same width as the ribs. The depth is ⅓ head from front to back. I draw the trapezoid shape from top of hips to crouch. I add my clay depth markers down the center of the stomach, forming those muscles to the belly button and the muscles below to the forming of the mons pubis. Then the lower back muscle markers are laid connecting the rib cage to the hip bone. Now the shape of the gluteus muscles and fat forming the shape of the butt, and I move down into the upper leg muscles and knee. The upper thigh from the side is 1 head at its widest, moving to the knee which is ⅓ of a head wide.

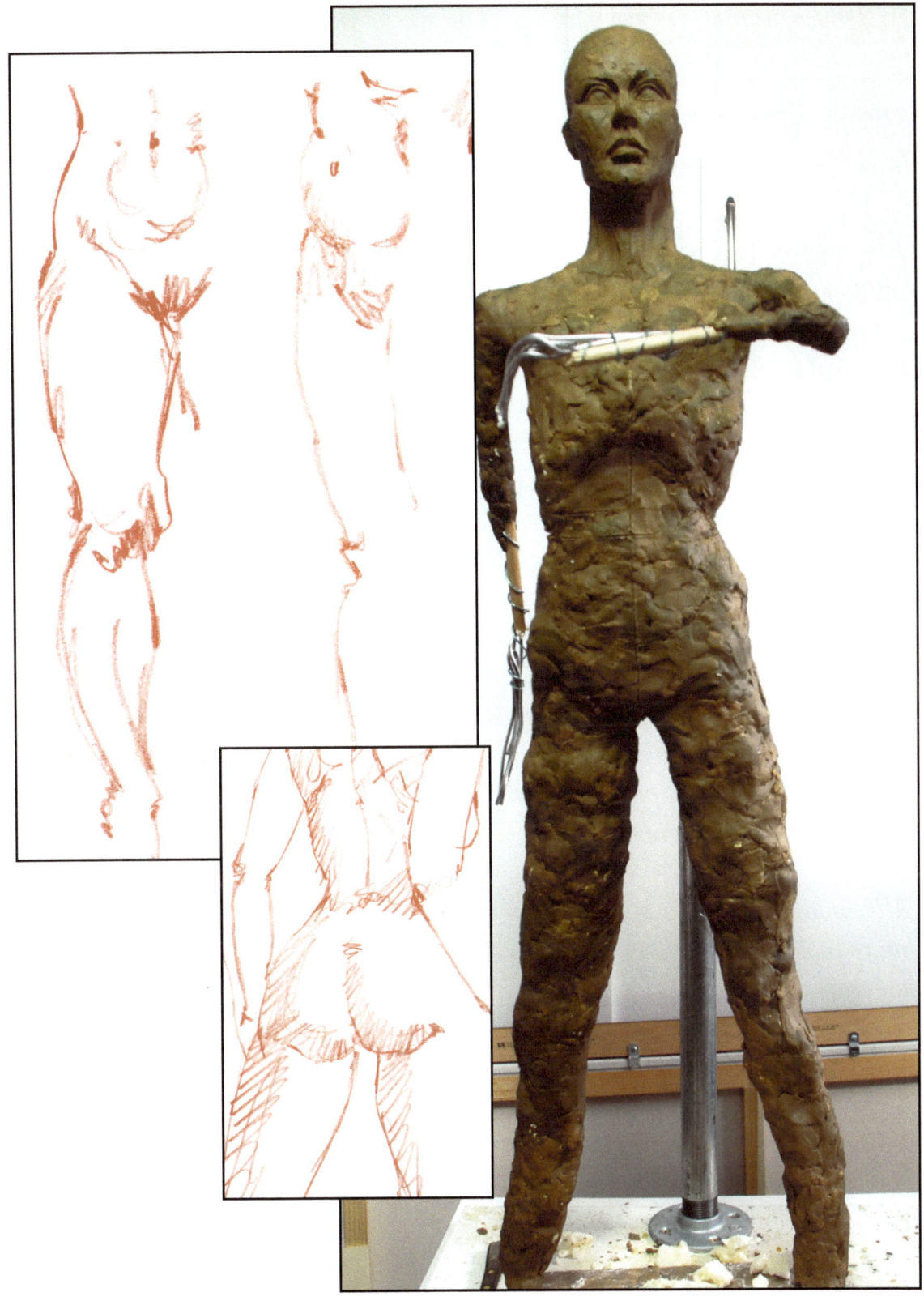

As I place the markers down the leg, it is ⅓ head wide at the calf slimming to ½ head at the ankle and moving to the foot which is one head in length.

Now that I have all of the markers laid, I add a ridge of clay connecting them from the side view only. Coffee break time.

When I return, I sit down and look at the figure from the eye level of the belly button. Taking my knife, I now re-shape the ridges to give them the shape of my "ladies". I have found that the math may be right, but that does not necessarily give me a figure I like. I trim down the muscles from the bottom of the sternum to the belly button and re-shape the muscles and fat forming the lower belly. I drop and curve the lower stomach muscle a bit, giving the figure a mature shape. Next I rework the shape of the back at the waist and add a smoother curve to the butt and drop it a bit where it meets the top of the thigh. I re-shape the leg adding more definition to the muscles and make them look like she is carrying her weight on the balls of her feet with the knees slightly bent. I sculpt and re-build the side view ridges to make them look correct to the size and shape of the head. I also have had to re-sculpt the head, making the back wider and a fuller neck in the front. The head is looking better as to the size and shape. All of these little changes to make it fit into one cohesive figure. Soon I will work on the markers for the shape of the figure from the front, and start to form the muscles, skin and finally the drape.

After many long weeks of working and re-working, I have finally found the figure that eluded me in my dreams. Her stance, curves and shapes, her presence, just from the side view alone, she is what her name promises. Tears swell in my eyes as I see my two sisters and Muzzy - warriors, standing to face the unknown with grit, determination, yet with softness and grace.

It's time to celebrate with Nancy, a single malt scotch for me and a Bailey's for Nancy, both in crystal glasses, and a toast to Connie and Muzzy, their memory will live on for millenniums, a legacy of courage for those fighting Cancer.

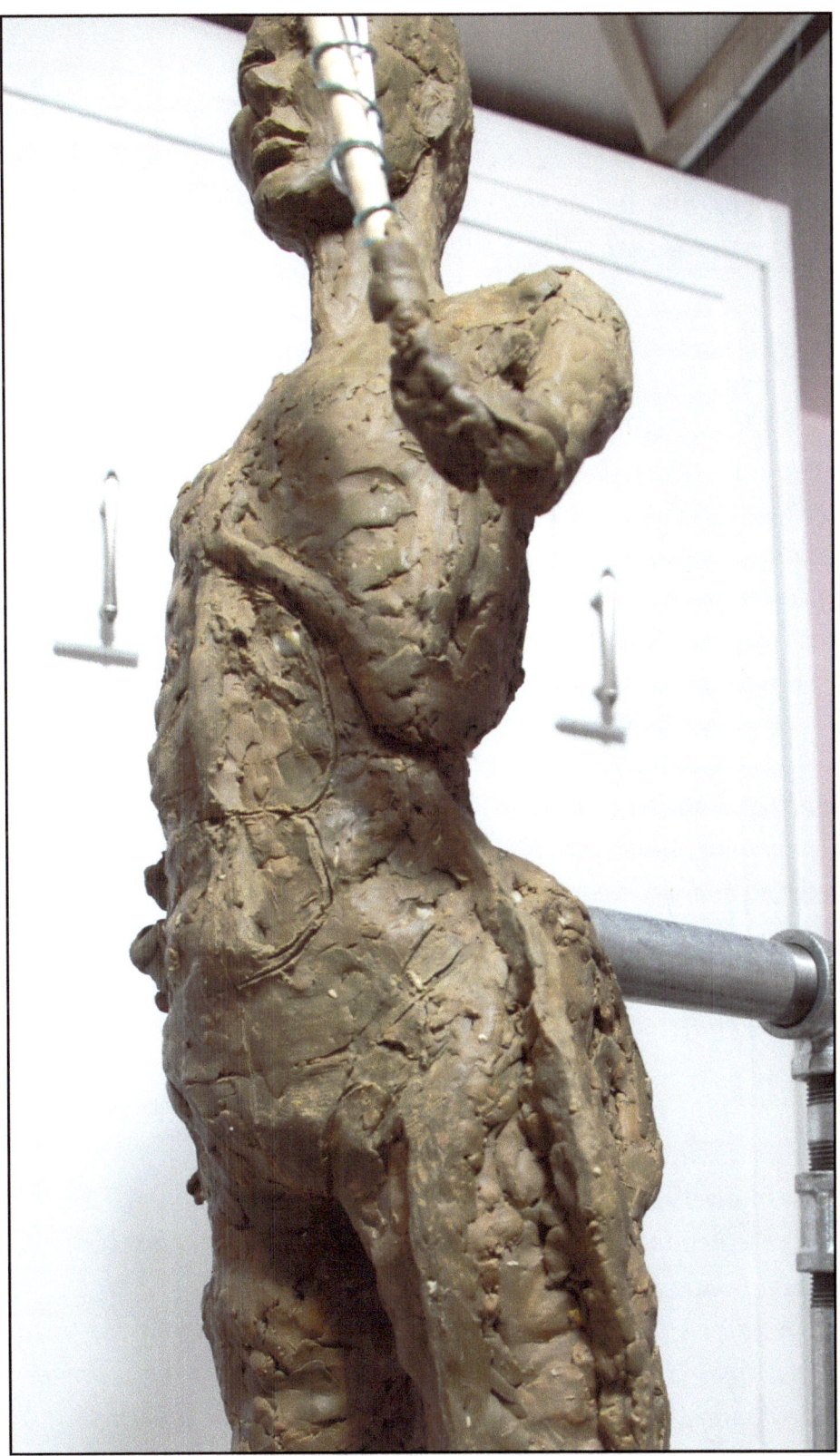

Maybe now no more dreams.

Nov. 25

I have spent a bit of time over the last few days building up one side of the front of "Courage", shaping and re-shaping the body so it works with the head. When I am happy with the shape, I will begin working all over the body.

The weather changed last night, turned chilly and raining. Our winter may have set in. My hands are rebelling. Because of the weather and the intense work with the hard clay this last week, my arthritis is screaming at me. My hands were in pain all night, so not much sleep. When I woke up this morning, my hands were so swollen I couldn't hold a pencil. So I put some hot water in a bowl and submerged my hands and rubbed them until the swelling went down and I could bend my fingers again. They are still very stiff and sore, but when I work in clay this time of year, that is what happens. Until they get better, usually when the weather changes again, I can only work a few hours a night.

Nov 28

The day after Thanksgiving, yesterday Nancy and I went in to Portland and had a holiday dinner with daughter Katie and Sam and Lexi, and Sam's parents. Good food, good company and uneventful drive there and back. Now today I will work on the entire body of "Courage". My hands are still sore and quite swollen, which is why I usually paint this time of year instead of sculpt, but this year is a bit different.

I have started filling in the muscles on the front since I have the ridges on one side to use as a guide. This includes shaping the muscles under the rib cage and the stomach muscles and building up the rib cage and shoulders. First I build the bones then add the muscles. I am having a problem with the top of the figure; since the head is bald the hair isn't there to add volume to the area above the shoulders. Because of this, the head looks too small in relation to the shoulders and chest, yet again the math is correct. I am spending a lot of time cutting down, re-sculpting the width of the shoulders (up to an inch on each shoulder),

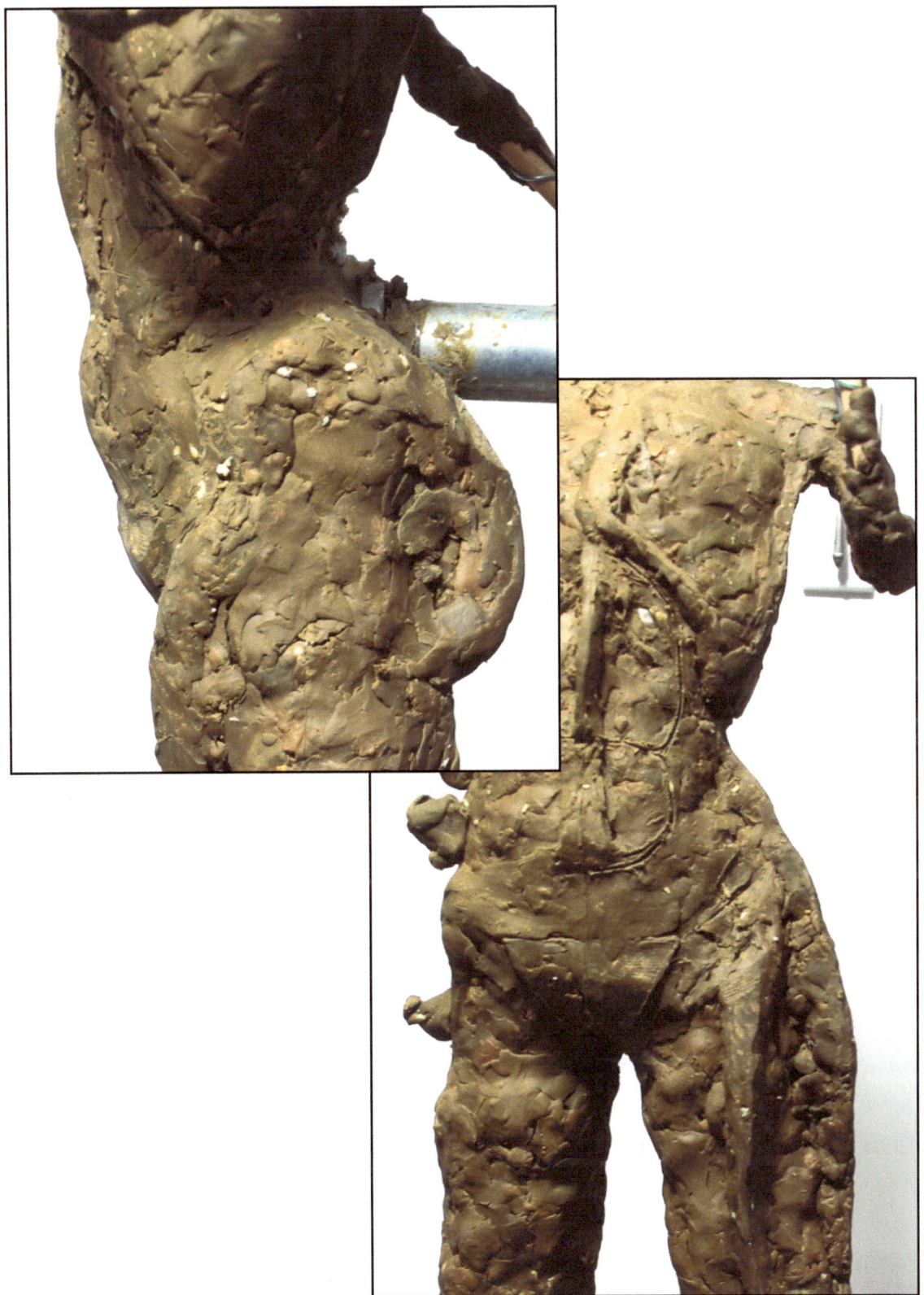

and rib cage, and also reworking the head shape to look correct. I've broadened the width of the face at the eyes and under the cheekbones, tapered the top of the head more, giving it a more elegant shape, and I have increased the depth and re-shaped the head from the ears back. The neck seemed too far forward with the new thrust of the body so I took some off the front of the neck and added fullness and a gentle curve to the back of the neck.

I got lost in my work again, in the zone as they say, the hours have sailed by. I have had the luxury of spending all day on "Courage" but now my body is rebelling. My back is screaming at me since I am constantly bending over the piece at odd angles. My shoulders are stiff and my hands have swollen up twice their size to the point I can't move them, time to call it a night.

Nov 29

Worked at the gallery all day and now after dinner I can again get back to "Courage". My hands will allow me to work a few hours tonight so I am lucky.

I want to accentuate her stance making her more tensed for battle, so I push out the base of the rib cage and rotate her hipbone forward adding more of a curve to her back also throwing out her butt more and moving the knees back. The legs I also spread apart a bit more at the hip, about an inch, but these simple moves have added so many more dynamics to the curves and movement that your eyes can now travel smoothly over the piece.

Re-worked her stomach, hips and leg muscles, by adding more definition to the muscles, she has become less "matronly" and more of my Amazonian style figure. By pushing her right arm back and behind more, her shoulder is now a good shape and her proportions look correct. Note to self: when I enlarge this piece the head form will have to be blocked in larger than normal and I will have to first work out the head and torso proportions to look right from below before I progress in blocking out the lower body forms. Nancy has looked at the piece and commented on "Courage's" big butt, so I went in and took off a few pounds, toned her up and made her curves a bit more flatteringly. Oh if it were only this

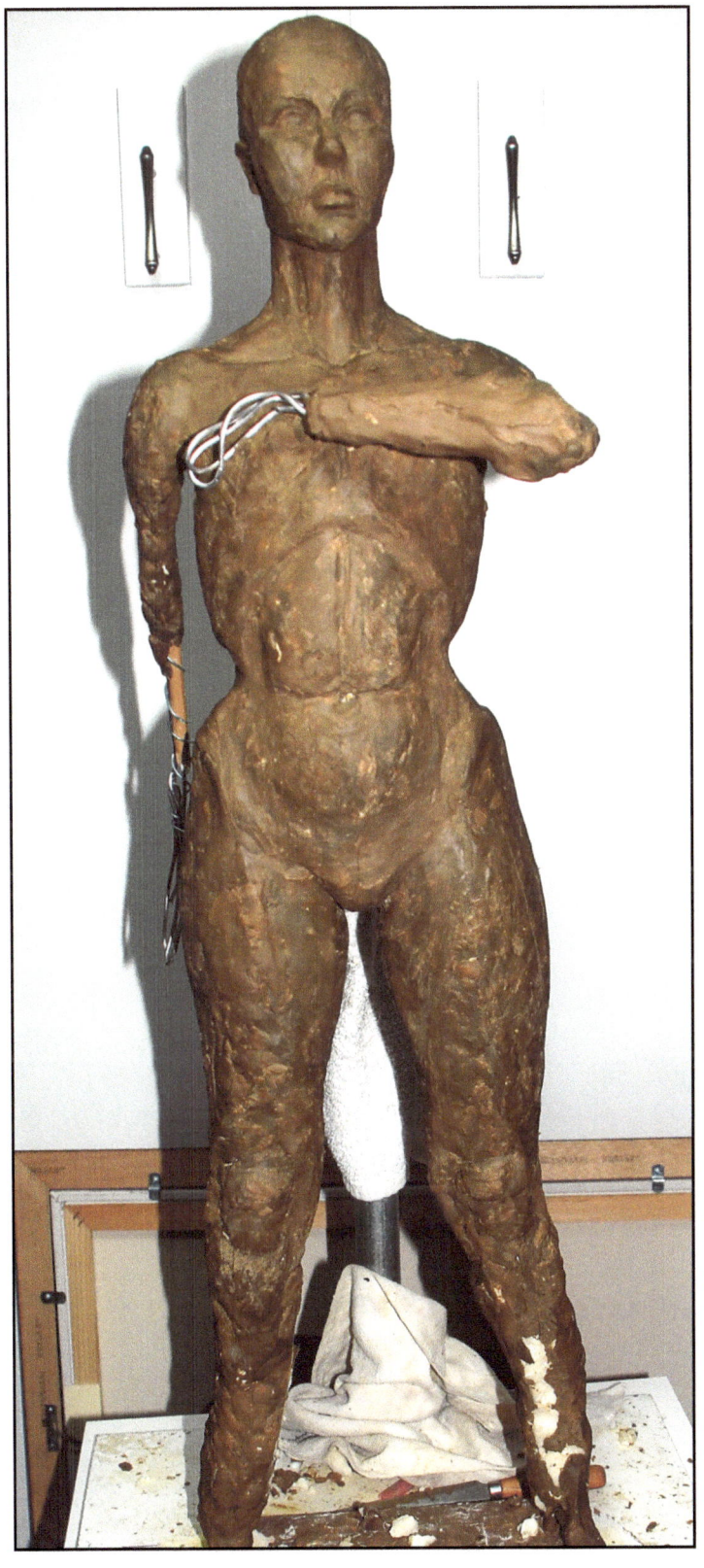

simple in real life to trim and re-shape our bodies. I'll take some photos from tonight and then off to bed.

Dec. 3

Today I want to start working on the drapery so I had Nancy pose with some different types of cloth and wrapped around in different combinations. The cloth that worked the best happened to be a long shawl. After about an hour, we got a wrap that looked quite good, and elegant. I took some photos of all sides then through the magic of Photoshop I cloned the drapery onto a photo of the clay "Courage". The next few hours were spent drawing and redrawing the drapery until I got what I wanted. A very simple drape, not too fussy, I don't want to see the drape first before the figure. So I simplified the folds, and made them hug close to the body. That is my sculpture style, the clothes meld into the figure, accentuating the muscles and form, and flowing with the figure, an impression of the cloth.

Dec. 7-11

I have been working on the drape; I thought I would cut some cloth and dip it in a plaster solution then wrap it around the clay figure. When dry, it would be hard and then I would add clay to build it up. Trouble was it became too fussy, too complex and too much attention on the drape and the folds. So I just threw the cloth away and started to work in the clay. Like the body I started with the markers for where the folds were. Then just started to drape the clay and make my own swirls to complement the flow of the figure. If you stop and study the drape, it might not make sense, but it looks right, is not the first thing you see or concentrate on and it flows with the figure which is all that matters. I start with what I know in all of its complexity then delete that which is not important and finally boil it down to its simplest form and action.

Dec. 12

Nancy went into Portland for a class yesterday and today so I have uninterrupted

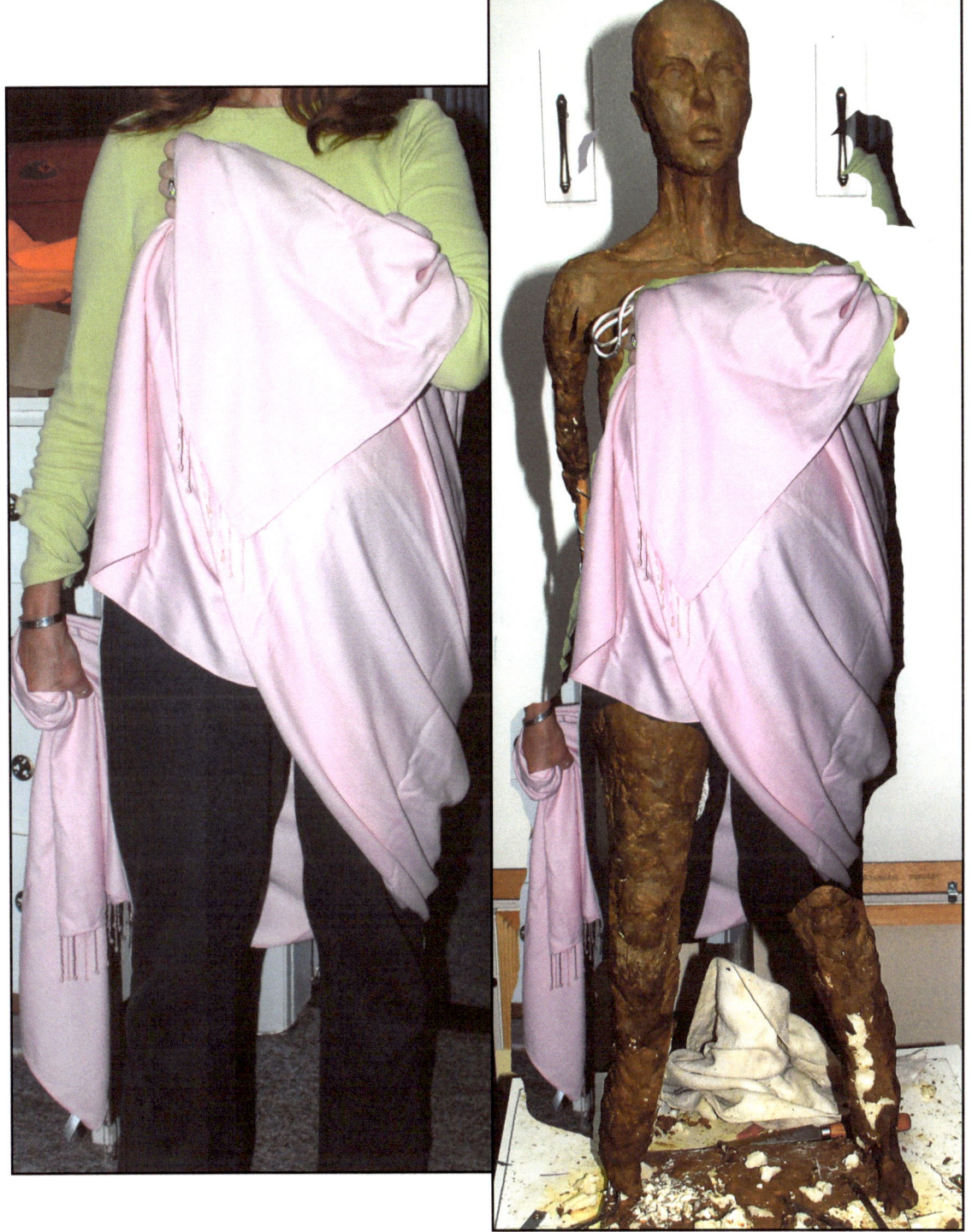

hours to work on "Courage". However a winter storm that hit us last night, took out a large tree behind the house which took out two power poles. No power today starting at 11am. I brought "Courage" into the front room which is all windows, western exposure to give me natural light. As the day gets on, the light fails quickly, so I get out the battery powered lanterns we use this time of year when the wind and rain blows from the north. We have sustained winds of 45mph and gusts of 70mph, and rain blowing in sideways. Forecast is for colder weather, high winds and snow on the beach on Sunday. Nancy will come home tonight over the mountains before the weather turns into a blizzard and she can't get across.

The drape is going quite quickly, as is the figure itself. I am not having the same problems I had with the head and face. The figure seems to be just coming from my hands and I am not spending a lot of time thinking about what I am doing. I am filling out the bulk in the rest of the figure in clay, and then I sit back and start to mold and sculpt the muscles. A curve added here and there to make the eye flow easier, move a muscle a bit to add to the tension and relax a muscle on the other side to calm the flow and give the eye a chance to rest before moving on to the next area of tension.

Dec. 20

I have been sick all week, what with the weather changes, cold snap, and temperature in the teens and even had 5" of snow on the beach and it has stayed all week. Travel treacherous as a second snow storm came through Oregon, Washington last night. Everything was closed.

A wonderful thing happened tonight; John called to talk about "Courage" and what was in the plans. He and Beverly are coming to Cannon Beach for the Spring Unveiling Weekend and the unveiling that Friday night of the finished cast piece of "Courage". He will buy the first 36" sculpture and donate it to the Summa Foundation Cancer Center at Akron City Hospital in Akron, Ohio, where Connie went to for all of those years, in her memory. They are building a new three floor center and John wants "Courage" in the entry way in the new

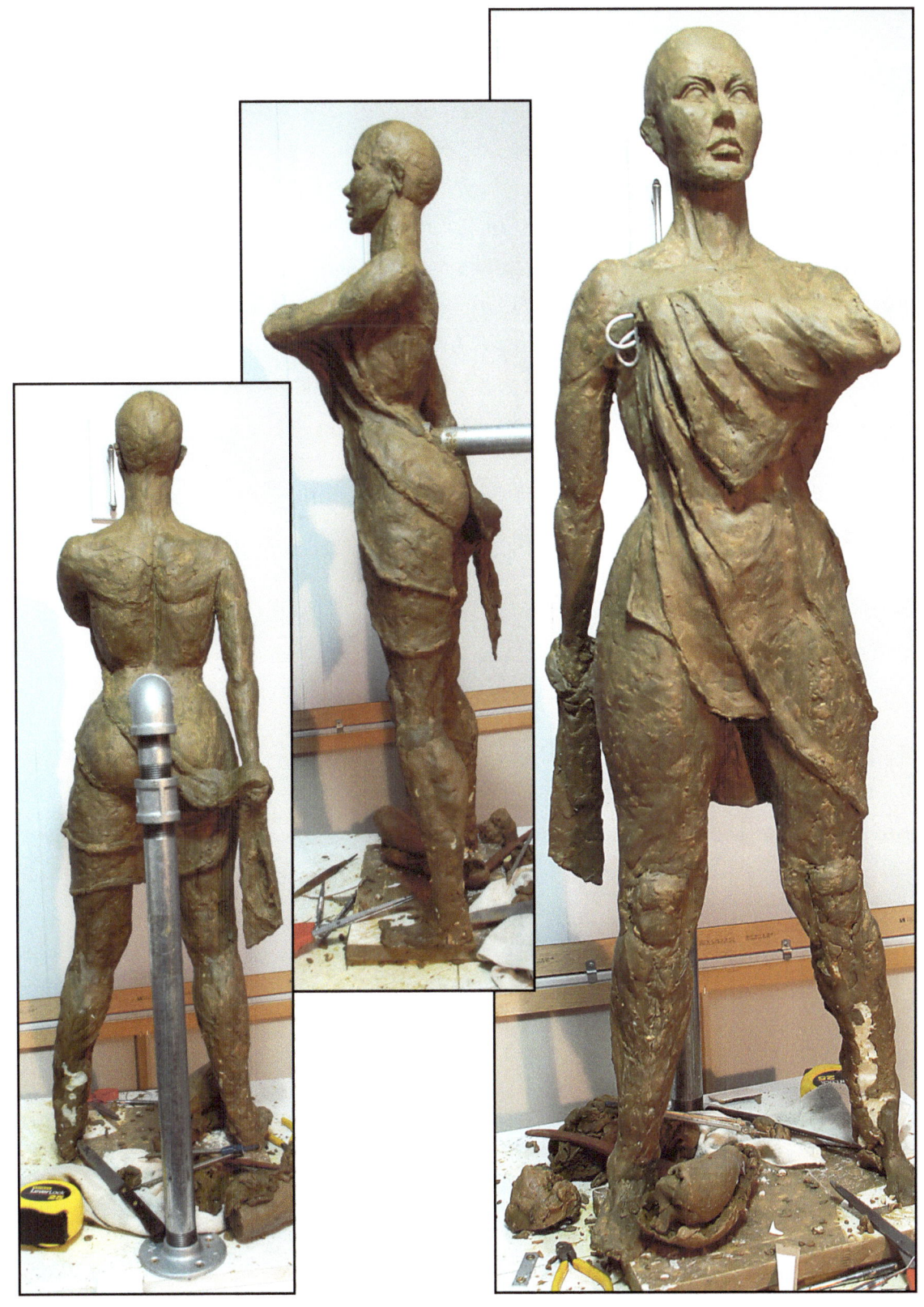

building for people to see and touch and find renewed strength and hope as they go to their appointments in the building.

We then discussed who he should contact at the Cancer Center to tell them about it, and how they should tie in an event with John presenting both the sculpture of "Courage" and a check for $5000 to Cancer Support Services. This fulfills the two purposes of "Courage". The sculpture is for strength and hope and courage, and the money for Cancer Support Services. This is a wonderful thing John is doing, and I can only think that maybe Connie has directed all of this, as her way of helping. We have come full circle, if not another sculpture is sold, she has fulfilled her purpose.

This edition of the 36" "Courage" will be #1 in a Family Edition, a special one not tied into the regular limited edition.

Now I have to finish the piece, hopefully by mid Jan., then off to the foundry for the final magic to happen.

Jan 2-6, 2009

A new year begins and "Courage" is kicking my butt right now. I have been working and re-working the drape on this piece for days. The drape is right, and the figure looks good, but the sculpture does not have the look and feel of my work. It is too smooth and there isn't a lot of movement to the piece. It is too static. Even though she is not passive nor does she lack power and presence, she still lacks the sweeping style and roughness of my other sculptures. I think at this point I need to take charge and make "Courage" the way I want her to be. I have allowed her too much say in the final stages; I need her to become one of my "ladies".

I start by tearing off the drapery and re-styling it, giving it a windblown look with swirls as well as folds. Without the hair and energetic movement of the limbs as in my other sculptures, the drapery has to carry the sweeping style and energy. The cloth starts to look like it is being blown by the wind from the front

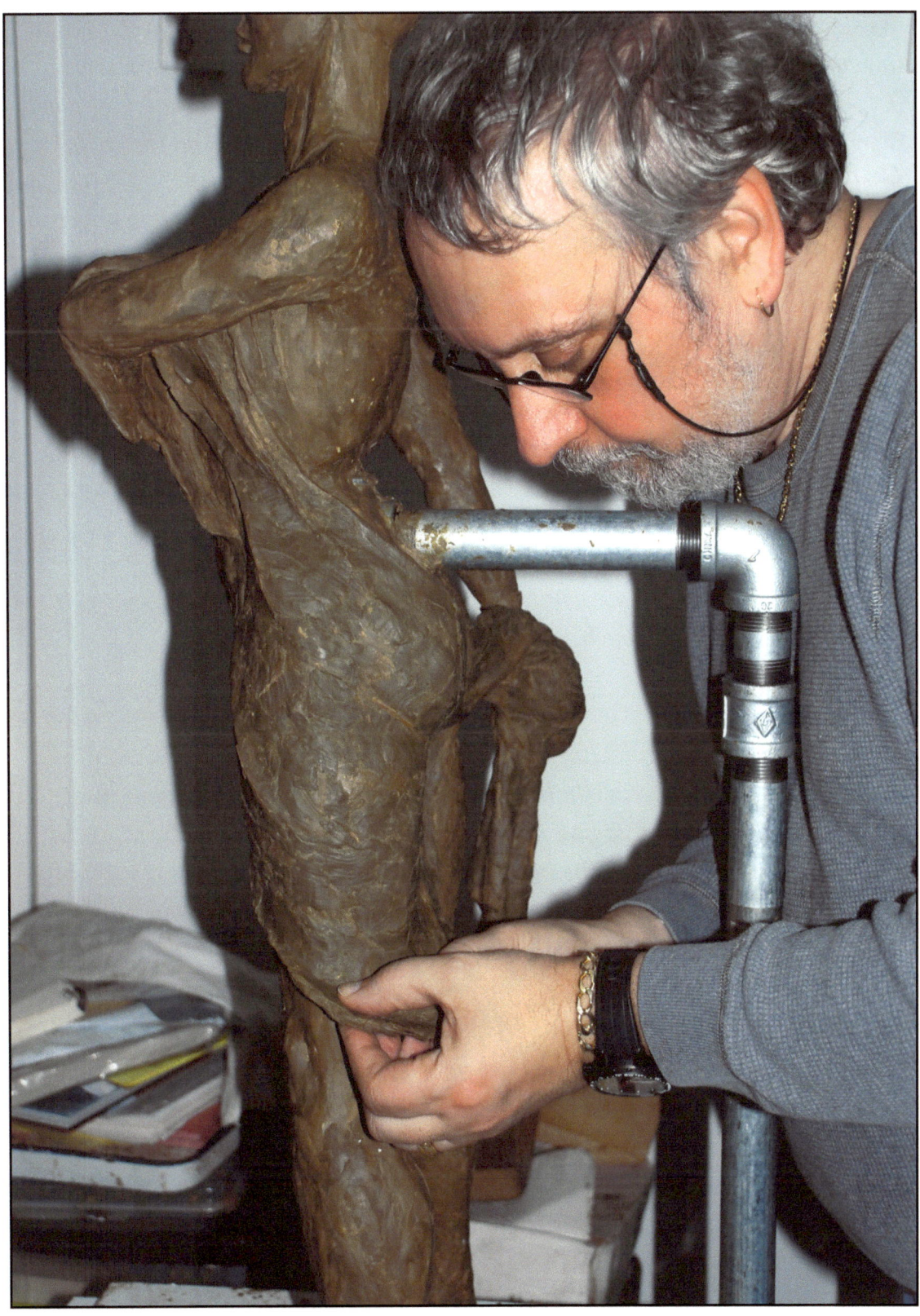

and side. A flip here on the side and it swirls around to a couple of deep folds in the back and gathered in a fisted hand. It now is looking more like a warrior, and the symbolism of a warrior; the texture of the drape on her body has a look of armor, the drape over her arm and hand could be a shield, and the shape of the cloth falling out of her right hand looks like it could be a sword. This is starting to have a lot of energy and depth in symbolism, and that is what "Courage" needed.

Jan. 10-13

I am adding the paintbrush impressionistic texture to the drape. Swish by swish, stroke by stroke, around and around the drape and body. "Courage" is now looking like mine. The rough texture of the cloth against the smoothness of the skin, the movement and energy as it swirls around her and gives her life and soul.

Jan. 14

The drape is finished, I have completed the butterfly necklace and bracelet, now the hands need the final touch.

Butterflies were a favorite of Connie's; she said they brought her peace, freedom and hope. At the cemetery after the internment ceremony, John who had bought several Mylar butterfly balloons, walked to the little lake alone and released the butterflies as he had promised her. We all silently watched as the wind suddenly came up and the butterflies took flight. Slowly they rose into the air and maneuvered themselves up and around the clouds, staying in sight and staying in the clear blue sky. Up and up they drifted. Nancy, my wife, walked over to stand with John as the balloons slowly left our sight and sailed to the heavens. So of course I had to have a butterfly on "Courage". Nancy and I joked several times that instead of a necklace, I should put a butterfly tat on her butt. Connie would have gotten a kick out of that.

As to why I added the bracelet? When my family heard that Connie's Cancer came back a fourth time and she was given six months to live, Nancy and I, Dad, Connie and John all met in Texas where my sister Beverly and her family

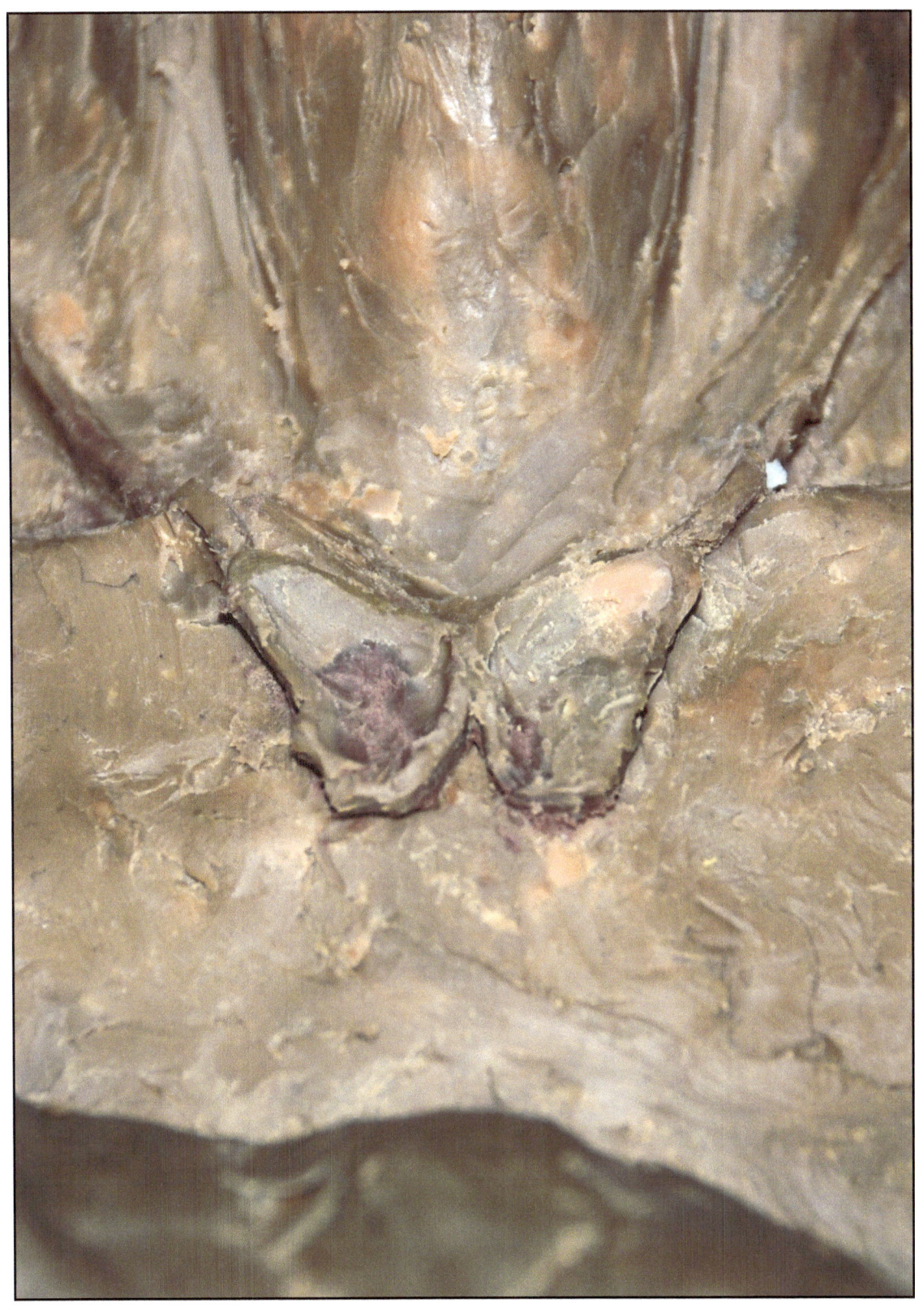

live. For a week we talked and laughed and reconnected. When Nancy and I left for the airport to come home, and I hugged Connie, I realized two things. I would never see Connie again alive and that the family needed something to help bind us together during these trying times.

I kept wondering what that something was, and finally settled on a bracelet. But what should it say? What can one say at a time like this? Nancy and I mulled it over for awhile, when I decided we needed to design a special silver bracelet and on the face it would say "Love Never Fails" from 1st Corinthians 13. Nancy went into Portland to a jeweler and had them design a simple silver bracelet with the phrase on the face and on the other side, the wearer's initials. Without saying anything to anyone, I had six made, one each for Connie, John, Dad, Beverly and Nancy and I. I then mailed it to each person.

When Connie died, John gave her bracelet to his daughter, Sarah, from his first marriage. She is a fine young lady that loved Connie as if she was her own mother, and Connie loved her as her own. A fitting gesture. To this day we all still wear our bracelets to help us stay close though we are thousands of miles apart.

That is why "Courage" has a bracelet that says "Love Never Fails".

Tomorrow I will concentrate on the left hand, the one holding the drape. Now it looks like a fist, it needs a softer more refined look. But not tonight. I have done all I can for tonight, I need a fresh look at it tomorrow when I can spend the whole day working on her uninterrupted.

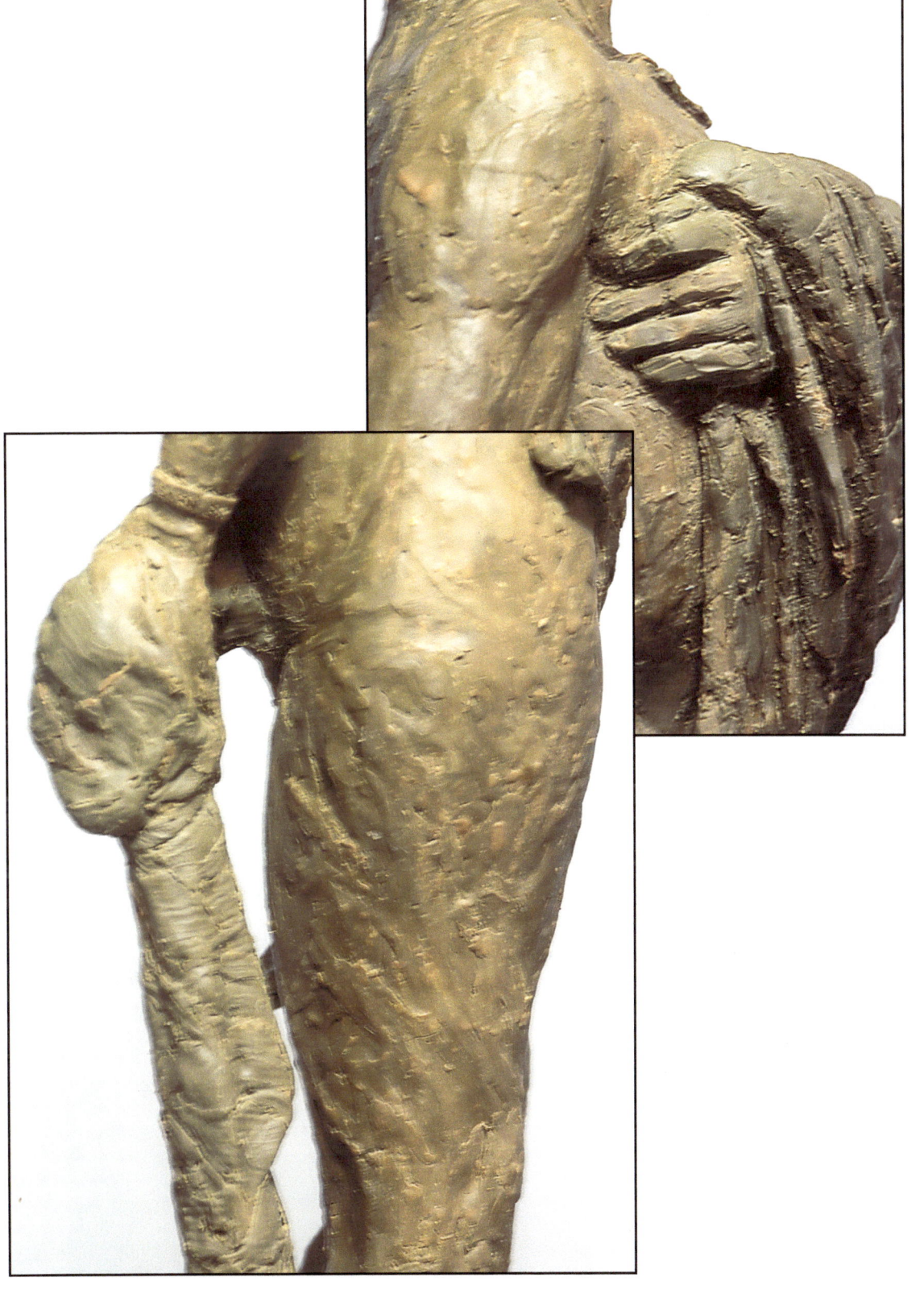

Jan. 15

Today I have completed "Courage".

She is all that I dreamed of and more. It was a struggle. It was painful both emotionally and physically, and yet it was a celebration of the lives of Muzzy and Connie.

When I finished, I took a long walk on the beach in the sun and the warmth and the solitude. The only sounds were those of the gently rolling surf and the seagulls.

When I retuned to the house, I sat on the deck, looked out over the sand and water, and smoked a cigar I had been saving for this moment, drank a scotch from a crystal glass then said a prayer of thanks to Muzzy and Connie.

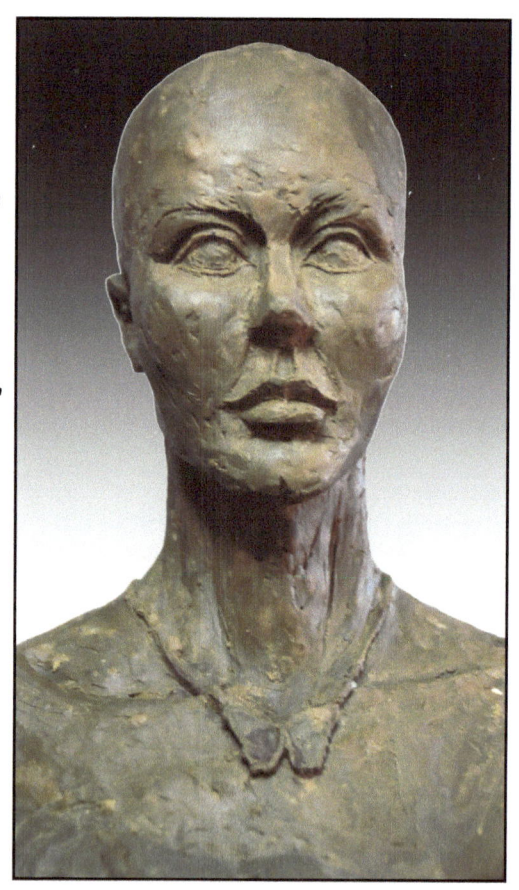

Thanks for the honor of knowing them and their gentle hands guiding mine. Thanks for their lives that have touched and enriched others. Thanks for the opportunity to help their spirit and courage live on and help others.

We all thank both of you for "Courage".

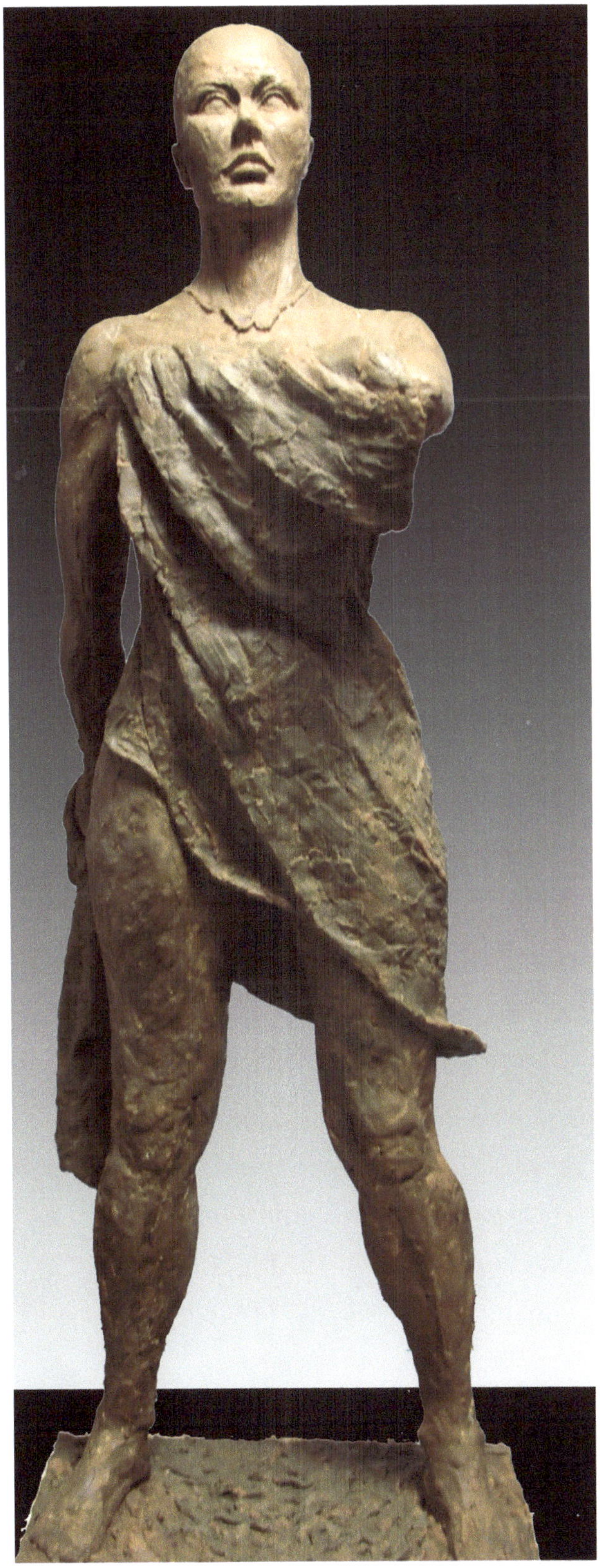

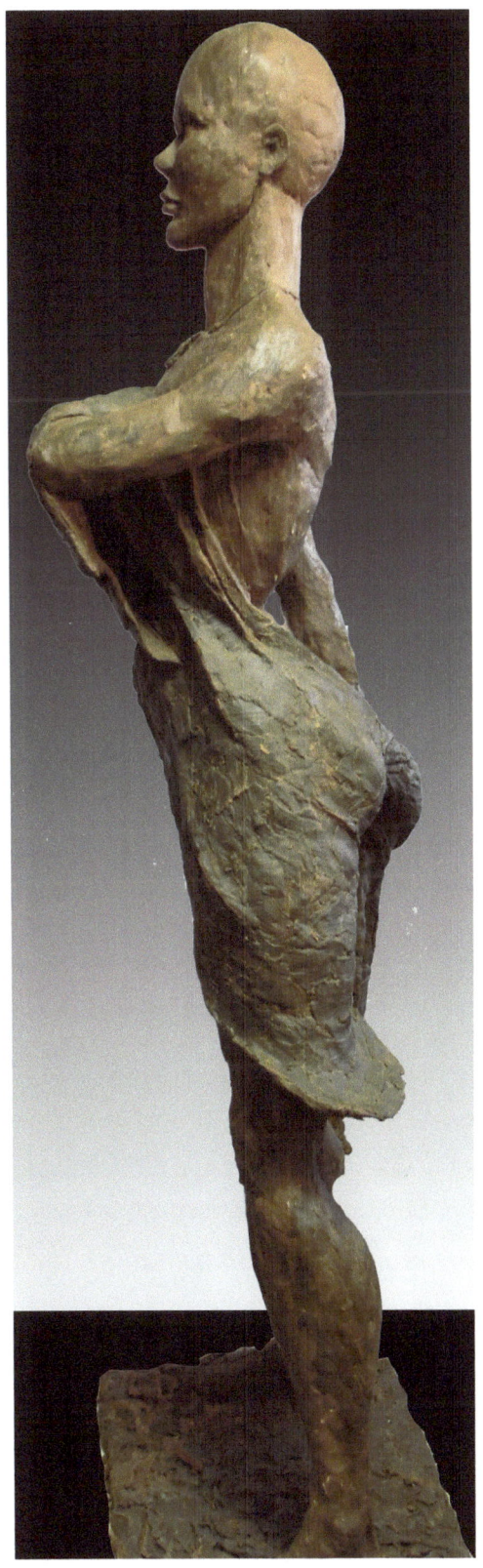

Here begins the foundry process of "Courage"

Some five thousand years ago during the Akkadian period, an artist carved an image in beeswax covered it in liquid clay and placed it in a hot fire. The wax melted out or "lost", leaving an empty space. Bronze - tin and copper - were melted together and was poured into the empty space of the clay. When the metal cooled, the artist knocked the clay shell from the metal. The first bronze was cast in the "Lost Wax" process.

Ancient "Lost Wax" bronze castings have withstood the centuries, and elements of the "Lost Wax" process have been refined over the centuries. Yet today, bronze casting in foundries is essentially the same as it was in 2,000 BC.

The finished clay model is cut into multiple sections

Step one is to saw apart the clay and wire sculpture, cutting into as few pieces as possible. "Courage" was cut into three pieces, each separate piece having its own mold made. The parts created by the molds will be welded back together and each weld painstakingly cleaned up to replace the detail lost by the mold making. I am not a part of this step. I drop off the finished clay and leave before the foundry makes their cuts. After spending all of those days building, I can't bear to watch the cutting.

Mold making

The original clay pieces are painted evenly with a liquid rubber (angelate), the same material as a dentist uses to make your dentures. When completed, the mold is opened and the original clay is removed. The rubber mold is made of half of the sculpture at a time. Notice the raised registration dots on the edges of the mold. This is to help align the two halves and keeping the mold in perfect alignment. "Courage" has taken on the look of a saint with the crown of dots and flanges around her head.

The original clay sculpture is undamaged and will be used as reference in the chasing steps to keep the wax and metal castings true to the original.

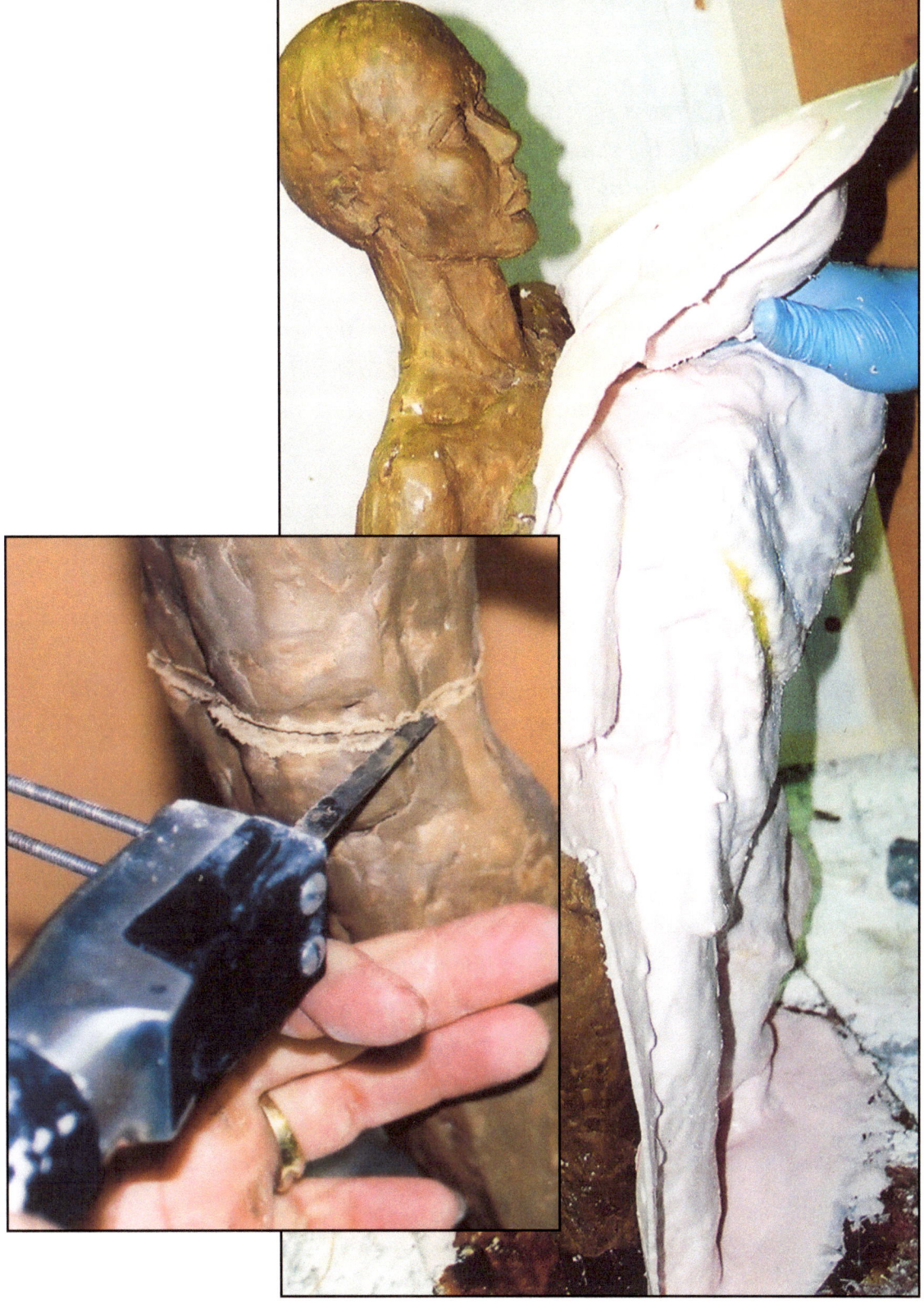

Creating the wax replica

When the rubber cures, a rock hard protective mold made of re-enforced plaster is built around the rubber. The mother mold halves are then put back together for the wax pouring. On "Courage" the face area in the mold was first painted with a thin coat of wax to pick up all of the fine detail of the face. Then the mold was put together ready for the wax pour.

Wax is melted, poured into the mold and evenly "slushed" inside. Slushing is repeated three times using cooler wax each time to avoid melting the previous coat. The wax wall will be about 3/16" thick —- any more or less might create flow problems for the bronze.

When the mold is opened and the rubber peeled away, an almost perfect wax reproduction is removed, then checked against the original clay.

The wax pieces are chased then applied to a tree

"Wax chasing" is the process of joining the wax pieces, removing seams and repairing imperfections by skilled craftsmen using heated customized soldering irons and dental tools.

I visited the foundry at this point to check the work and integrity of the wax pieces. I had two sculptures made and in checking, I found that one gave me goosebumps when I saw her but the other one did not. Carefully I looked at the face of the second one and found that it was not quite right. The mouth was "off". It was lacking the curled smile that I realized was my daughter's smile. This was the first time I was aware I had added her smile.

The foundry repoured the entire wax piece since we knew the mold was right. When I held the new wax, I again got goosebumps ... the smile was right.

"Vents" (thin wax sticks) and "gates" (thicker wax sticks) are affixed to the wax

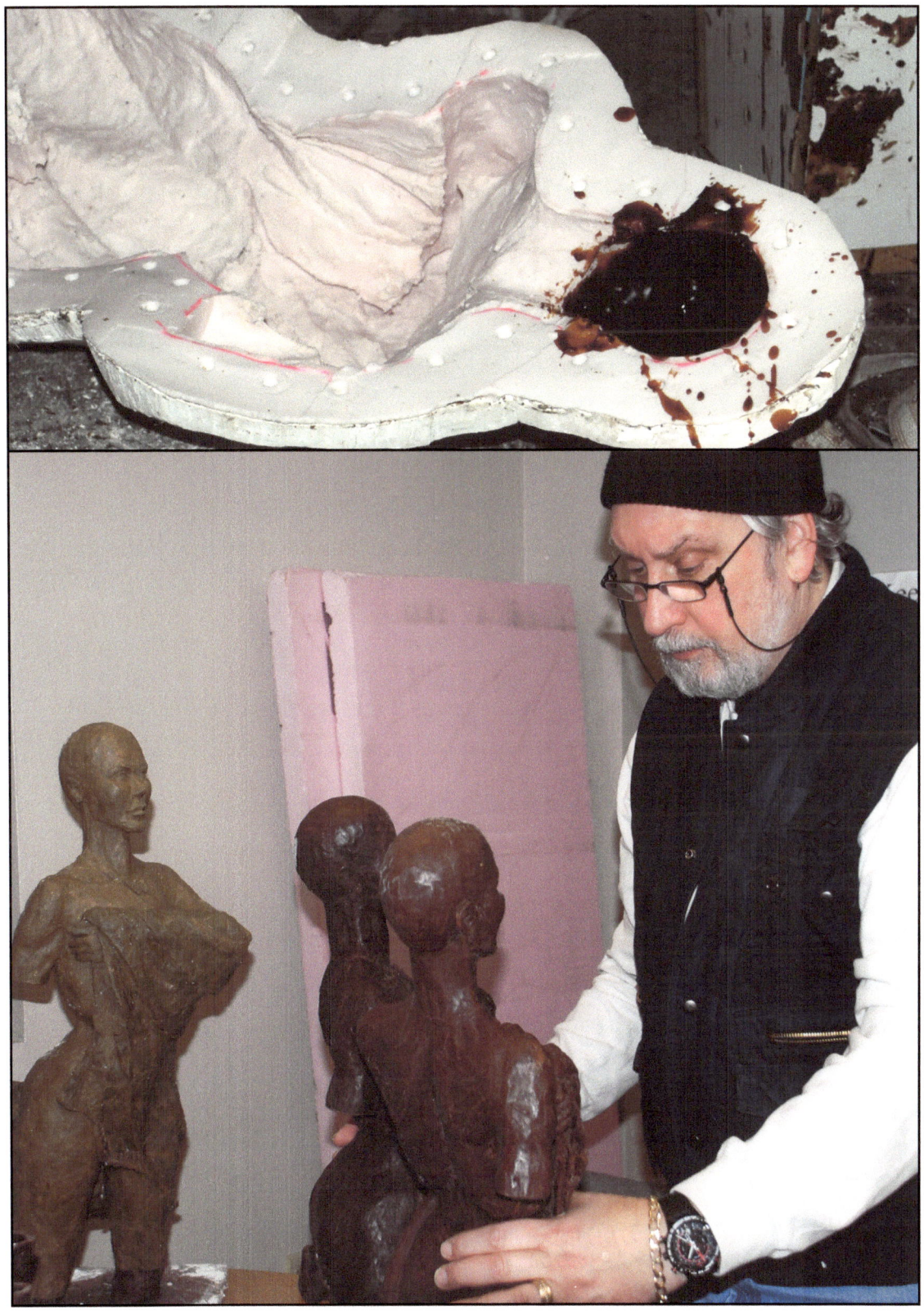

reproduction forming the "tree". In the casting process, the space occupied by gates becomes runways through which the metal flows and trapped gas escape.

Ceramic Shell

The next step or "Investment" is the process of building a hard shell around the wax sculpture. When the wax has been melted out, the investment will serve as a mold for the hot bronze.

The building of the ceramic shell begins by dipping the gated wax or tree into vats of slurry followed by sand. This process builds a very thin wall of silica around the wax. The process is repeated once daily for approximately two weeks, or until a hard shell about ½" thick forms around the wax.

The phrase "lost wax casting" comes from the wax being melted or "lost" from the ceramic shell. The shells are "de-waxed" in a high pressure autoclave; plaster invested shells are still de-waxed in a kiln.

Pouring the Bronze

This is the "Show" of the making of a bronze. Here I am going to revert to technical verbage from several sources on the internet since I can't think of an easy way to give you the info. Here goes.

A graphite crucible is filled with bronze ingots that are melted. The metal melts at 2000°F. Bronze stops flowing when confronted with cold, which might occur if molten bronze was poured into a room temperature shell; so at the same time the bronze is being melted in a furnace, the ceramic shell is heated in a kiln to approximately 1100°F (see the photo on the right of the glowing shells).

When the "Dance of the Pour" begins, the crucible is lifted out of the furnace. At the same time, the glowing ceramic shells are brought out of the kiln to the pour area. Two artisans operate the crucible in a "jacket." The artisan with the controls is the "lead pour," the artisan maintaining the crucible balance is known as the "dead man." A third member of the pour team the "safety" pushes away dross and slag on the surface of the molten bronze.

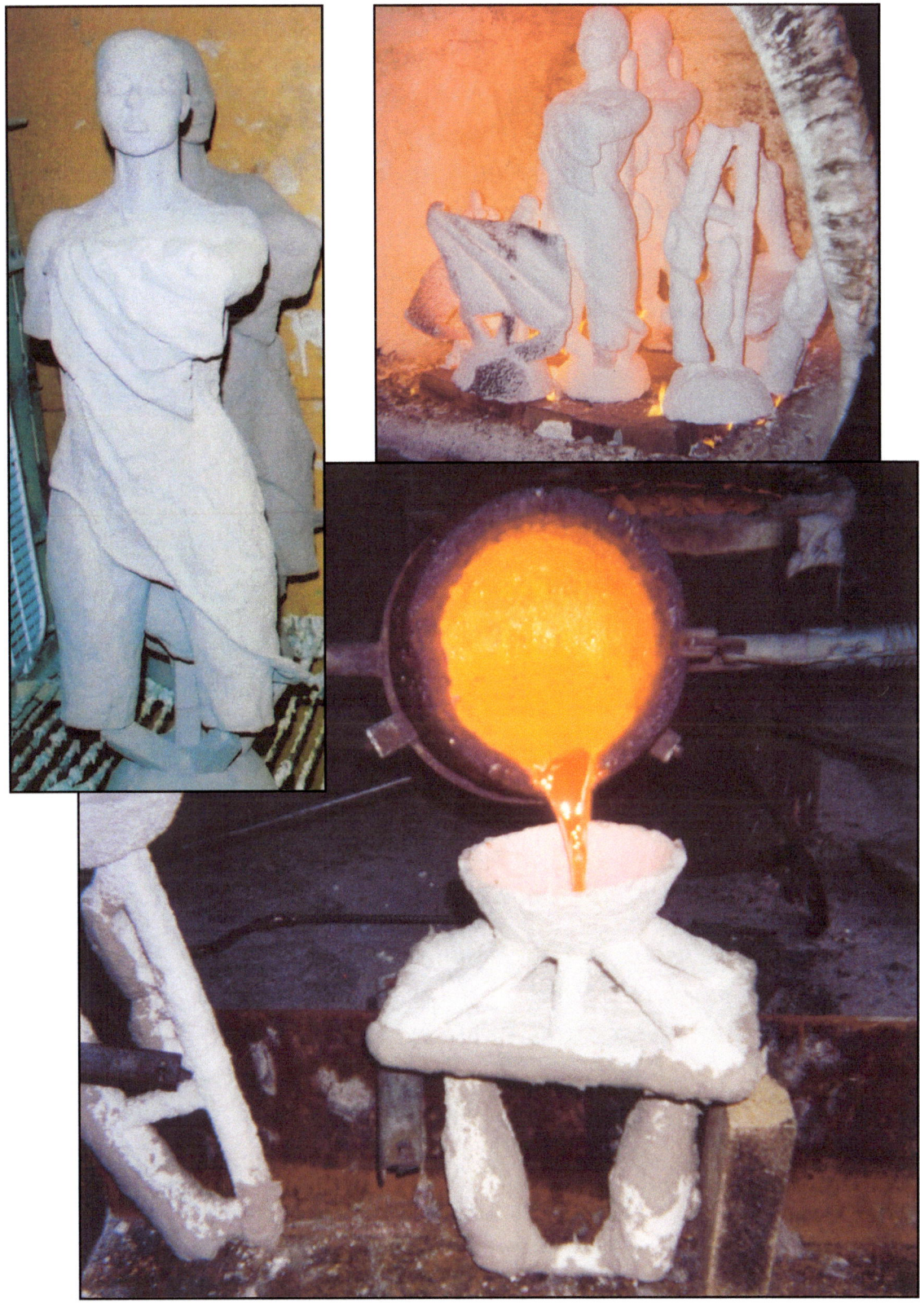

The entire pour is very fast and very precise; one crucible of bronze holds 140 lbs and can fill one or two medium shells or ten or more small shells. The first pieces poured are those with thin walls and intricate details; requiring hot, fluid bronze to move throughout the channel system.

Silicon added to the bronze helps the "flow ability" of the bronze instead of using lead or tin. A modern day addition to the centuries old process.

Removing the ceramic shell

Removing the shell from the metal is called "Devesting". When the piece is cool enough to handle, hammers and power chisels and a lot of skill are used to knock the investment off the solidified metal. The gates and sprues are removed with a high intensity electric arc that can cut through the bronze like butter.

Welding, chasing and sandblasting

After the three sections of courage are welded back together, the bronze must be chased to take down weld lines formed by the joining of two planes and to fill in the slight imperfections.

The chasing starts with large electric or pneumatic grinders to remove the bulk of the unwanted metal. Then, more refined and smaller tools such as die and pencil grinders are used to re-create the surface texture.

Before going to the patina area, the casting is sandblasted to remove any fine investments from the bronze. Notice in the photo above the tin color of the finished sandblasted bronze next to the original clay pieces. Here is where I come back to the foundry and check the metal against the clay to make sure it is correct. With these two sculptures I had done, one of them was leaning forward a bit too much, so she went back to the metal area to be cut apart above the ankles and re-welded to stand more upright.

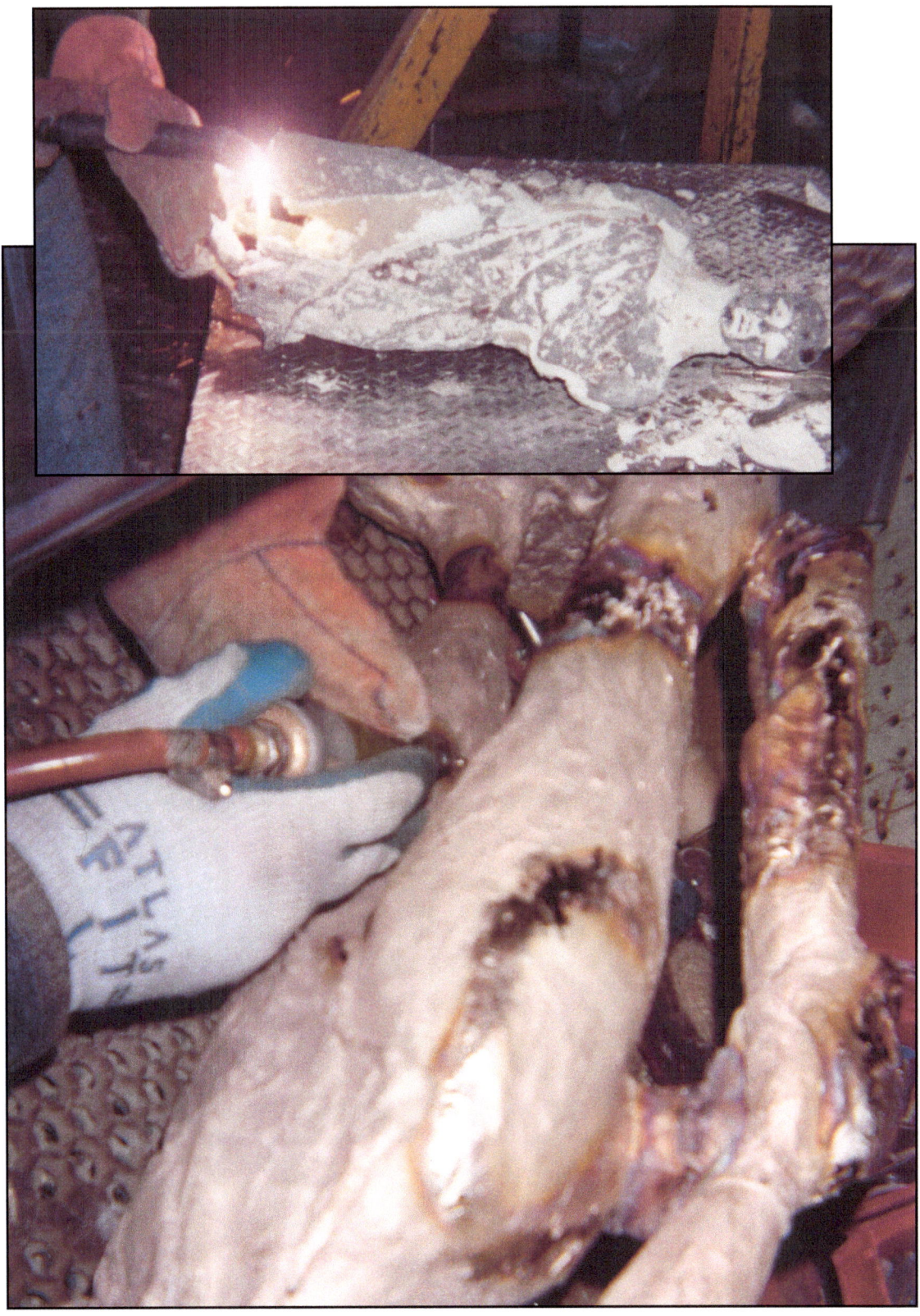

Patina, final finishing and assembly to base

This is the anxious part for the artist. The patina is the enhancement of bronze by spraying chemicals on the hot bronze for the color. There are three water soluble   compounds that form the basis for most patinas and I used two of them for "Courage". I originally wanted a light tan sculpture instead of my usual "Classic" colored pieces. The foundry cast the hand and cloth piece for me and tried a white/tan patina for me to look at before the whole sculpture was cast. I didn't like it, and they did another patina test. It was not the right colors for "Courage". The colors were too light and ethereal looking and "Courage" needed to be strong and grounded, a warrior with presence. So back to the "Classic" bronze color. Ferric Nitrate was applied first to produce the classic reds and browns. Notice in the photos that a blow torch is used to heat up the metal and the chemicals are sprayed on and set with the flame. I want the color of the piece to have a depth of colors so the chemicals are applied then rubbed off a bit then more applied and so on until the colors are right. I wanted the piece to look a bit aged so a slight dusting of Cupric Nitrate was added to create the greens. Take a close look at the last photo on the right. The patina work is finished and now it is time to apply the hot wax to seal the colors. Here the green color which was   applied last disappears into the browns when hit with the hot wax. Magic and the patina artist knowing what the end result will be, irregardless of what it looks like before the end.

After putting the thin coat of clear wax over the bronze to enhance and preserve the patina "Courage" was screwed into the granite base and her journey came to an end.

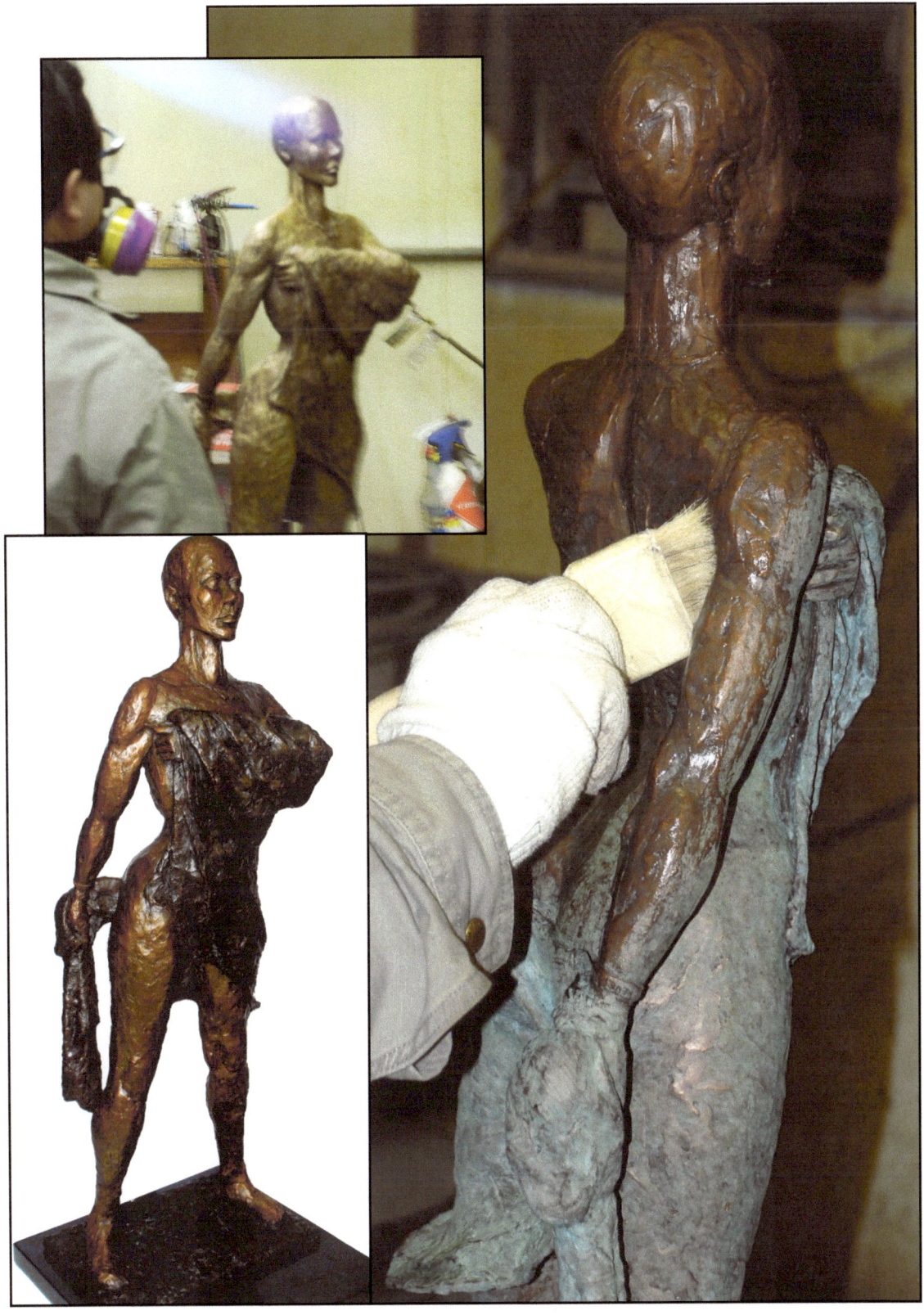

About The Artist

Michael Tieman was born in a small town in Iowa in 1950, but his family moved every few years around the mid-western states. Thanks to the encouragement of his fourth grade school teacher, Michael picked up a charcoal pencil and started to draw. For the next eight years, he filled his evenings and weekends taking art classes to round out his art education, including watercolor and oil painting, sculpture, printmaking, pottery, and his first love drawing.

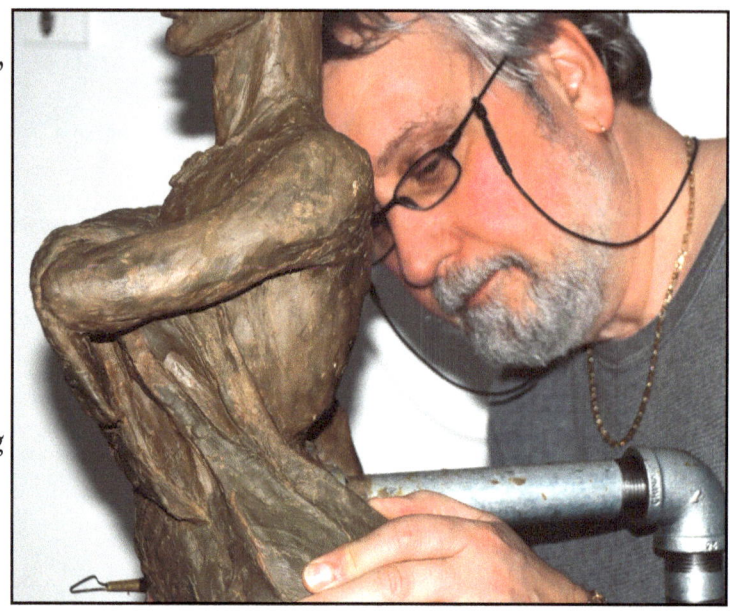

In 1968 Michael attended the Columbus College of Art and Design in Columbus Ohio and in 1972 received his BFA.

Taking his degree, Michael and his Canadian wife Nancy went to Vancouver B.C., Canada where she worked as a dental hygienist and he started out on a successful thirty plus year career in advertising. The years passed quickly with working and raising two wonderful daughters, Heather and Katie.

After completing Expo 86 as the Sr. Graphic Designer, Michael relocated in 1986 to Portland, Oregon with his family. Nancy taught clinical dental hygiene at Oregon Health and Science University while Michael worked in several ad agencies.

In 1993, Michael opened MT Studios in Portland, an outlet for his fine art. In 2001, thanks to the encouragement from his family, Michael put his advertising career on hold and devoted his time and energies toward paintings of the Pacific Northwest's landscapes, seascapes, and people.

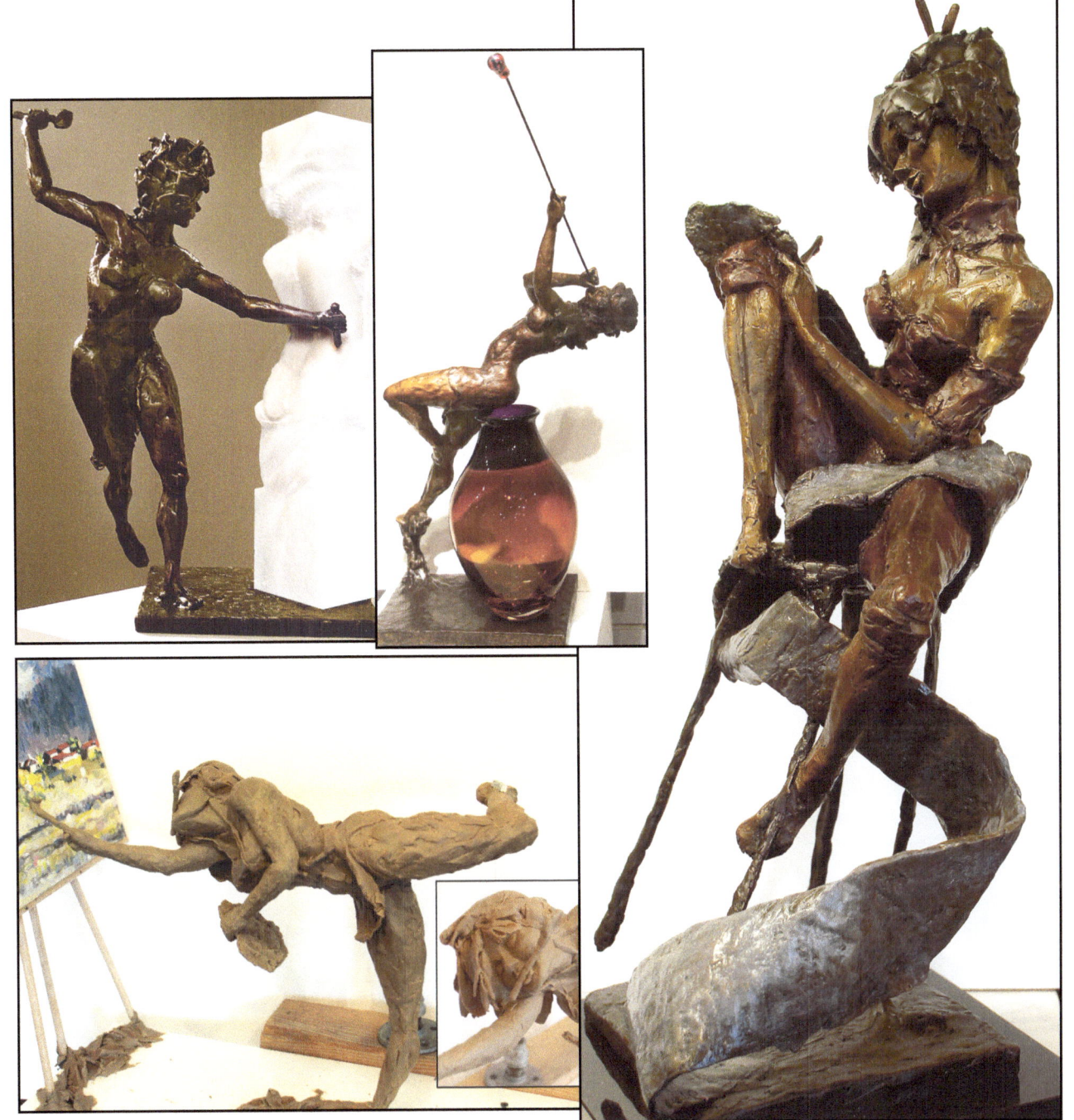

Clockwise: "The Stone Sculptor", "The Glassblower", "The Poet", and "The Painter"

The uniqueness of the "Hands of the Artists" collection, is that the final sculpture includes two complete works of art, the Artist and their Creation. I am sculpting the artist at work on their creation and that figure will be cast in bronze. The second piece, the Creation will be an original one-of-a-kind piece, usually done by another artist.

The "Hands of the Artist" collection is dedicated to several unique art disciplines: The Glassblower, The Stone Sculptor, The Poet, The Painter, The Weaver, The Photographer, The Potter – Wheel, The Potter – Raku, The Wood Carver, The Jeweler, The Dancer, The Clay Sculptor, The Musician, and The Blacksmith.

Each year Michael Tieman plans to release two new Artists in the collection. They are cast in bronze, in limited editions of ten each.

"My work is a combination of all of the techniques I have employed over the last fifty plus years in graphic design and fine art. In painting, I am concentrating on the medium of acrylics on canvas, refining my "early impressionistic" style of thick bold strokes of colors, strong abstract design, movement and texture, impasto over washes, and accents in the primary colors."

A year later, Michael and his wife Nancy, sold their house and cars, packed up their "kits" and settled on the Oregon Coast in Cannon Beach. Here they opened their own art gallery, Artists Gallerie, a dream Michael had for 30 years. Artists Gallerie was not only an art gallery which represented a dozen artists, but it was also Tieman's studio.

"The role of an artist from the dawn of time has been as a visual storyteller. The stories my paintings and sculptures tell are ones of confidence, strength, passion, playful sophistication and the celebration of life."

Following the encouragement of a friend and gallery owner, Michael in 2003 expanded his artistic talents into sculptures cast in bronze. Tieman's sculptures are unique in that they are a combination of traditional figurative sculpture and his Impressionistic painting style.

"I create my bronze sculpture as a three dimensional painting; texture is the impasto brushstroke, color is the play of light and shadows across the surfaces, and detail is the free style movement of the impressionist style."

Michael is the artist in residence and showing his paintings and sculptures at Haystack Gallery in Cannon Beach. Nancy is pursuing her education and passion working as a mental health therapist with teenagers in the county.

Tieman is a member of; Pacific Northwest Sculptors, International Sculpture Center, National Sculpture Society, Oregon Society of Artists, and the Cannon Beach Gallery Group – (Board Member since 2002, President-2005 & 2008), and is currently writing a monthly column in the local newspaper.

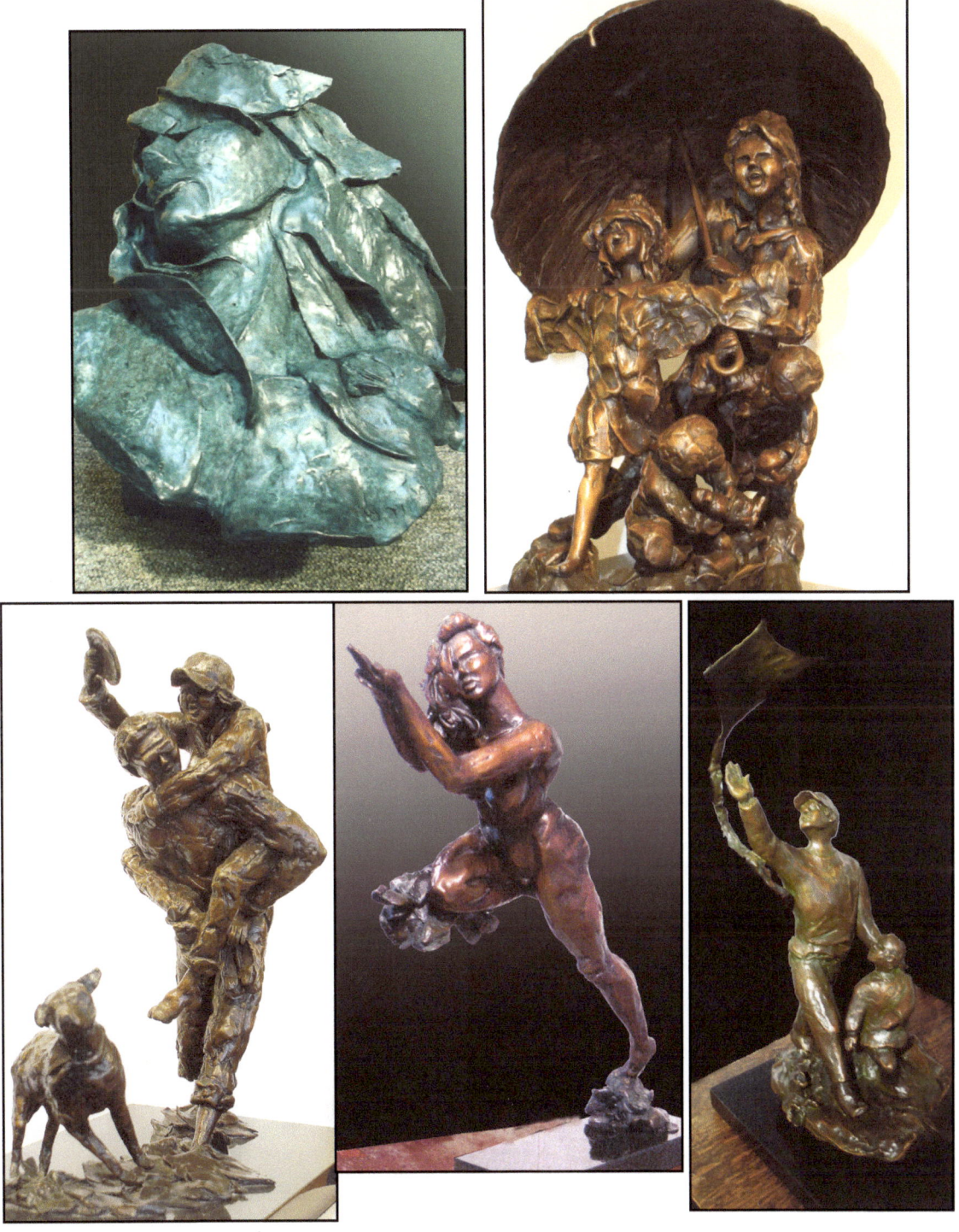

Top row, left to right: "Spirit of the Sea", "Playing in the Rain"
Bottom row left to right: "Surf Play", "Behold the Gift, "Let's Go Fly a Kite"

My Thanks

Thank you Nancy for staying by my side for almost forty years. You are my soul mate, my wife, my rock and my sanity.

I want to thank all of those who shared their stories and opened themselves up to me. I know how hard it is to talk about the pain, the anger and finally the knowledge that it is better now for your loved ones. I listened to you, made some changes and "Courage" is stronger for all of your input.

My friend of many decades, (far more than we want to admit at times), Steve, who has kept me questioning. We push each other and our abilities, thanks for his tireless work to get this book produced.

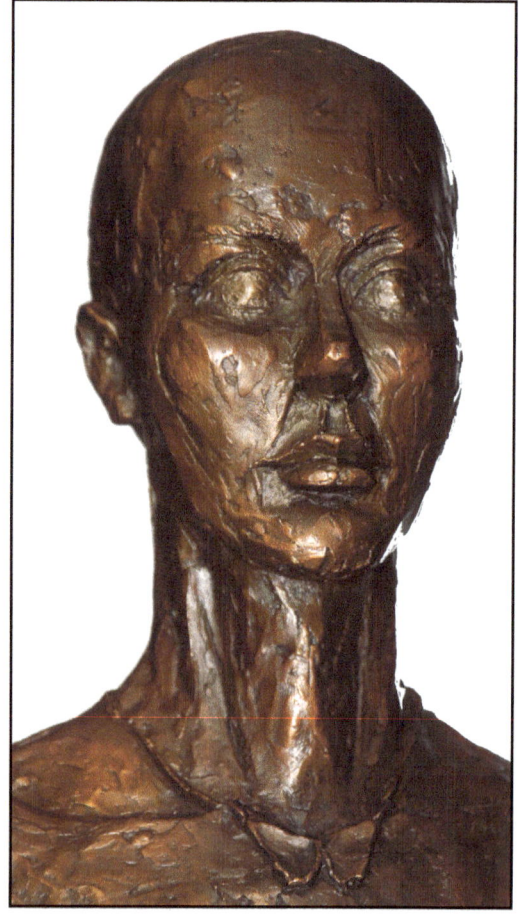

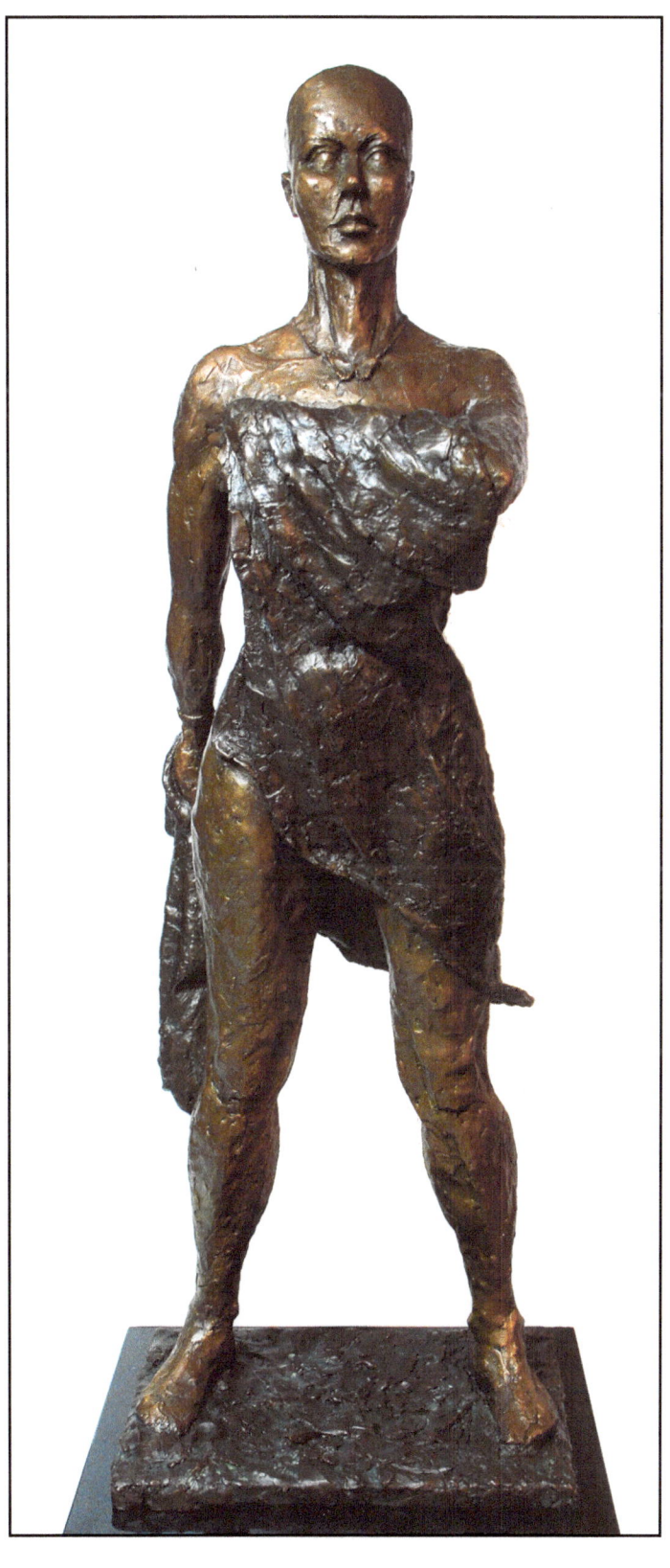